Breathe

Believe

Become

LIVE YOUR BEST LIFE NOW!

MARY CAROLINE CRAIG

LIVE ALIVE FIT
Living your best life...Alive, Healthy & Fit

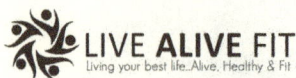

BREATHE BELIEVE BECOME

Publisher's Cataloging-In-Publication Data

Live Alive Fit

Breathe Believe Become: Live YOUR Best Life NOW!

Mary Caroline Craig. -1st ed.

Issued also as an ebook.

ISBN: 978-0-9961874-1-1

Printed in the United States of America

*This book is dedicated to those who bravely go after their dreams to live the lives they deserve, despite fear and resistance. Anything is possible when you **Breathe, Believe, Become.***

ACKNOWLEDGMENTS

*For my daughters, Alessandra and Bella,
who constantly remind me to be present
and* **BREATHE.**

*For my husband, Jay, who believed in me
before I could* **BELIEVE.**

*For my dear friend Debby Stinson, who taught me that
through sharing love, you* **BECOME.**

I am beyond grateful to have found my true passion in life. I get to share what I know with so many others who desire the same. Thank you to everyone along the way who supported my journey to health and inspiring others.

I would especially like to thank Hal Marshall, Beth Kozura, Christine Trainer, Anna Gurnhill, Joslyn Hamilton, Danielle Zissou, Dr. David Maxwell, Dr. Brian Krabak, Transformation.com friends, and many others without whose loving energy and support I would not be who I am today.

For my beautiful extended family, Mother and Father. You continually inspire me to keep moving forward in the direction of my dreams. Thank you.

CONTENTS

FOREWORD

As a sports medicine physician and an athlete myself, I have been fortunate to take care of athletes of all ages and abilities. My experience as a physician has allowed me to work at the highest level of competition involving professional sports and the Olympics. My experience as an athlete has helped me understand the importance of movement, patience, dedication, training, and perseverance. All these experiences have shaped the care and counseling I provide for my patients on a daily basis. And if there is one thing I can appreciate, it's that with an open discussion of life's goals and challenges, everyone can succeed.

But let's face it, that's not always an easy task. Sometimes you need to take a few steps backwards to appreciate how to move forward. (BREATHE) Ever watch a professional athlete train or compete at an important race? All athletes know how to focus on the task at hand, shutting out surrounding distractions. This may occur through a variety of techniques including relaxation exercises and positive thinking. Athletes use visualization to show themselves how they will succeed. They BELIEVE that all their hard work and training will allow them to achieve their goals. (BECOME) Sometimes it works and sometimes it doesn't. But they learn from both their successes and failures, correcting what is needed in order to try again. And hopefully enjoy the journey.

It is with this perspective that I hope all of us can learn from Mary Caroline Craig's wisdom. As one of my own patients, I witnessed firsthand how it took Mary an open discussion, some self-reflection, and a catalyst in order to spark the internal fire needed to help her start her transformation without excuses. It was slow, frustrating, and challenging. But her success stems from her ability to starting believing in herself, taking control of her surroundings, and developing a team in the process. She didn't need to be an elite athlete—most of us aren't. But we all possess a drive to succeed, if we can just find it. So in the words of one of my favorite lead singers...

"Dream up the kind of world
you want to live in. Dream out loud."
~Bono

...and Breathe... Believe... Become.

Brian J. Krabak MD MBA FACSM
Sports medicine physician and Olympic doctor at the
University of Washington's and Seattle Children's Sports Medicine Center

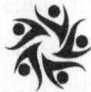

How to Use This Book

Be Patient and Kind

Lasting change takes time, and so can the achievement of big goals. Taking small steps, one after the other, can bring momentum that cannot be underestimated. Remember to pick yourself up, try again, and keep forging ahead in the direction of your dreams. We all deserve to have a fulfilling life—one that we feel embodies us and our true spirit. Realizing where we are at now, choosing what we want for our future, and taking the steps to get there takes time and hard work, but it can be simple. **Breathe.**

One Step at a Time

Most of you will benefit from reading this book all the way through first, and then going back to read one chapter every few days. As you do so, take the time to thoughtfully answer each of the questions in the action steps you will find at the back of the book and on my website. By following this process, you can focus on the specific steps you need to begin fulfilling your goals. Taking it one step at a time will generate a belief in yourself and create the desire you need to make your goals come to life. Let's get going. **Believe.**

I Am All In

You may already be motivated to make changes in your life. If so, you can begin reading and answering the questions in the action steps from your heart. The steps can be printed from my website at www.livealivefit.com, or you can find them in the back of this book. In this way, you can begin moving in the direction of your goals and dreams right away. Seize the day. **Become.**

INTRODUCTION

Many people talk about living the life of their dreams, but don't know where to start. They want to make life changes, but don't believe it is possible.

Well, it is.

I know because I have done it myself, and if I can do it, so can you!

Today I am a competitive multi-sport athlete, a wife, and a mother of two young girls, and I work full-time as a speaker and integrative health coach. I understand that balance in life is key. Even with limited time, I know that it is possible to make great changes in your life while still being present with your family and friends. After all, I did.

Six years ago, I lay in bed, recovering from three slipped discs, with sciatic pain shooting down my back. I was hardly able to walk. I decided I didn't want to live a life of despair, physical pain, and defeat any longer. With hard work, belief, dedication, and the motivation to feel strong again—both inside and out—I began to see a light at the end of the tunnel.

- ❀ I fully recovered from spinal injuries without surgery.
- ❀ I became eighty pounds lighter and learned to curb my emotional eating.
- ❀ I transformed my relationship with my family.
- ❀ I began walking, then running.
- ❀ I competed in marathons.
- ❀ I redefined my relationship with money and my finances.
- ❀ I learned to swim at age 38.
- ❀ And I started racing triathlons (swim/bike/run) and duathlons (run/bike/run).

Just eight months after learning to swim, I competed in my first IRONMAN® 70.3® triathlon. One year later, I finished the 140.6 mile IRONMAN® [1] Canada, Whistler Triathlon. Those races weren't even on my bucket list when I was lying in bed, but I did them, because I could!

One year later, I qualified to be a member of Team USA in the ITU Age-Group World Championships in Spain, and will soon be representing Team USA again in Australia.

I could hardly walk six years ago. Now I am a full-time health, nutrition, cycling, and triathlon coach; a certified yogo instructor; as well as a competitive world class age-group Duathlete!

I have gone from self-pity to enjoying every minute of life. The best part is that I now get to help others find and go after their true passions in life, while enjoying more health than they could have even imagined.

Everything in my life changed because I took control, set achievable goals, and went after them. Along the way, I gained more clarity about what was truly important in my life. Despite my busy schedule, I now spend quality time with my children and husband each week.

I have learned to live fully in the present by releasing control of things that aren't mine and letting go of things from my past. I am truly LIVING my life, not just letting life happen to me. I have a sincere passion for life and a love of people.

I believe it is possible for anyone to live their best life. With dedication, hard work, belief, accountability, and motivation you can reach goals you currently think are out of reach—with laughter and fun along the way! No harm in giving it a try, right? What is the worst that could happen? You could actually achieve a goal you have only dreamed of! So join me.

It is YOUR turn to...

Breathe,

Believe,

Become!

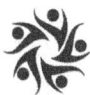

SECTION ONE

BREATHE

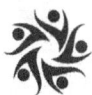

"I simply do

What many dream of.

I simply do

What others talk about.

I simply become

What others dare not

Even to imagine."

~ Sri Chinmoy

TAKE INVENTORY

*"Sometimes the questions are complicated
and the answers are simple." ~Dr. Seuss*

W hen I think of the word *breathe*, I think of slowing down: hearing and feeling my breath. I feel quiet, calm, and at peace. But it wasn't always that way.

For some of us, stopping to breathe means having to take a closer look at ourselves when we'd rather just keep powering through life and ignoring those things we do not like or wish were different. Slowing down, for many, brings on fear of a loud, cluttered mind full of negative self-talk. But if you are reading this now, some part of you wants to stop, breathe, and reconnect with yourself.

Slow down. Take a deep breath. Give yourself a moment to stop and think.

How do you feel? Energized? Tired? Joyful? Sad or depressed? Content? In love? Overwhelmed? Alone?

Are there areas in your life that you don't pay attention to in hopes that things will work themselves out on their own? I know I've been guilty of this, but is it working for *you*? If not, you may want to rethink your strategy. If you feel lack in any area of your life, you shouldn't continue to overlook it. If you continue along in the same direction, you won't be pleased with yourself five to ten years from now.

NOW is *your* time to take control of *your* future. Make a conscious decision to live—not on the sidelines of life, watching the game go by, but *in the game*, taking charge of each move you make.

> *"Fear is excitement without the breath."*
> ~Robert Heller

Is it going to be easy? No, but it can be simple. As simple as looking at where you are, where you want to be, how you want to feel, or what goal you want to achieve—and then creating a plan to get what you want.

When you take it step by step, you will hardly believe how much closer you are than you ever imagined to achieving some of your greatest goals.

Life is funny that way: when we truly want something, with all of our heart, and when we are passionate about it, make it a priority, and go after it, we usually get it.

I did, and you can too.

Life Can Change in an Instant

Each of us has a story—a very important story. You may not realize it now, but you have value. We each have something to learn from one other as well as from ourselves. I feel so strongly about this.

I have shared with you a bit of where I was and where I am today, but now I'd love to tell you how I got here. Why tell you my story? I want you to know that you are not alone. Even when facing emotional, physical, financial, or other challenges, there is hope and the possibility of living your best life.

I was a healthy child who loved to dance and sing and play, and so I had a full, exciting childhood. My life was filled with loving family, great friends, good food, and the inspiration to go after my dreams.

Then, in my early teens, I suffered a low-back injury while dancing ballet and tap, followed by a knee injury while running track. I stopped running, but continued to dance. The art of dance brought me joy and gave me an escape from the challenges of college. I loved being on stage and felt it was the one true place I could share my feelings with the world. Although my back gave me trouble from time to time, it always seemed to get better eventually.

After college, I met my husband, and we quickly became good friends. He and I shared our thoughts, dreams, and insights into life. We laughed a lot and enjoyed skiing, camping, dancing, and singing with each other. We looked forward to an active life together.

But less than one year after we were married, we were rear-ended on the freeway. Although our car was towed away, we seemed alright. I went to sleep that night shaken but hoping for the best. What I didn't know is that when I woke up the next day, my life path would be forever changed.

It was a Friday morning. My alarm went off, and as I tried to roll over to turn it off, something was terribly wrong. I couldn't move. I had suffered severe whiplash and upper spine and neck injuries in the accident, and after having suffered from low-back pain for the previous ten years, I was worried. My husband helped me out of bed and to the doctor. I couldn't turn my neck, could barely hold my head up, and needed help doing everything from dressing to brushing my hair and teeth. My husband couldn't even hug me without causing me to feel pain. This was serious.

The discomfort was terrible, but the humiliation was worse. I had to ask for help doing almost anything. I lost my job because I couldn't type without pain. I had never been fired from a job before, and I felt cast aside and angry.

A few years and many doctor appointments later, I was starting to get my life back. There were always going to be visits to my chiropractor and massage therapist, but I had escaped a huge blow with what I thought was minimum residual damage to my body. I knew one thing for sure: I wasn't going to allow my injuries to define me. With optimism, I began taking yoga to strengthen my core and spine. I wasn't sure I would ever dance or ski again, but maybe I could at least stay relatively healthy.

What I didn't know then is that our spines have histories, too. Once you damage them, they are never the same.

My husband and I had a good marriage. But after the birth of our first child, I found that I had a series of new problems. It began with constant infections that my daughter and I gave each other while breast-feeding. I felt guilty for having to give her medicine and guilty for eventually no longer being able to breast-feed her. Soon, I was taking medicine for postpartum depression, too. I felt sad and lonely even with my family by my side.

With a history of depression in my family, I was worried. I chose to throw myself into work, opening a floral and gift store when my daughter was eight months old so I wouldn't have to think about what was going on in my head or body. I had gained forty pounds from emotional eating and wasn't sleeping well.

The lack of energy and weight gain continued, and keeping myself busy wasn't masking the pain I felt inside. Despite all the work I had done to heal my back, I still had constant pain and could hardly enjoy time with my new daughter.

After some self-reflection, and increasing back pain, I knew I had to do something different. I attempted to take small steps to move myself forward. My goal was to lose some weight and get off medication. I opted for a diet plan with weekly check-ins, and like the good student I am, followed all the rules, learned to limit my calories, and eventually became lighter. I felt more present and was able to stop the depression medication. However, the diet did not teach me to exercise or eat quality foods, so it was just a small step.

My husband and I decided to try for another child. I got pregnant, but miscarried several weeks later. I was devastated. How could this happen to me? Was I being punished for something? Even though I already had a beautiful daughter and a husband who loved me, once again I felt sad, alone, and misunderstood. I threw myself back into work and tried to move on with my life. I never let myself grieve or truly deal with the pain.

A year later, I gave birth to our second daughter. I found myself again needing to lose a little weight after she was born, but this time kept the depression at bay. We decided to close my flower shop so I could spend more time with our daughters. Soon I was pregnant again, but once again miscarried. This sent me into a deep depression. I gained fifty pounds and started to feel pain in my spine again.

I knew I needed to become lighter, work on feeling better about myself, and get back to exercising. To begin moving again, I chose a group Pilates class. Surrounding myself with others who wanted health, in a class setting, gave me the accountability I needed to move forward. The core- and spine-strengthening exercises were just what I needed to relieve pressure on my back. Within a year, I became lighter, stronger, more confident, and in control—something I hadn't felt for years.

Then, after months of feeling better, I woke on Christmas morning with pain in my right calf. I didn't think much of it at first, but over time both my calf and lower spine hurt more and more. Once again, I couldn't move easily, and in just six weeks I gained twenty pounds. I wasn't able to sleep more than a few hours a night, and turned to sugary foods for comfort.

One morning I woke up and simply couldn't get out of bed. I knew it was serious when my trusted chiropractor insisted I needed an MRI on my spine. I could see in the technician's eyes, and hear in his voice, that there was a serious problem, but only a doctor could provide a diagnosis. He gave me the numbers of two spine specialists to call right away. I left the office with scans in hand, then sat in the car and cried. I thought my life as I knew it was over.

The first available appointment with a spine specialist was the following Wednesday. I drove gingerly to the appointment, my right calf cramping, unable to turn my body much at all. It took me a long time to get from car to office. The walk to the front counter seemed to take an eternity.

After checking in, I found a wall and waited; sitting was not an option. When I was called back, I was embarrassed to be in my mid-thirties walking like an old lady. I used to be a strong and beautiful dancer. I used to fly through the air with ease and grace. Now I was fat, depressed, and hobbling down the hall, holding onto the walls to steady myself.

Just breathe.

When I entered the exam room, I saw autographed pictures of successful athletes lining the walls. I later learned that my doctor was both an endurance athlete and doctor for U.S. Olympic teams. I was humiliated to look the way I did, but he was kind, patient, and caring. He examined my spine and leg, looked at my MRI scans, and told me what I didn't want to hear: my L4, L5, S1, and partial S2 disks had slipped out of my spinal column and were being compressed into my low back. The disks were pinching the sciatic nerve running all the way down my right leg to my calf. There was no way to fix or move them. Pain management would be my new life.

I felt as if I had been handed a life sentence. My days of skiing, dancing, and simply living a normal life seemed to be over. I began intensive physical and occupational therapy just so I could get through my days. Small steps would move me forward.

It's time to believe.

My first physical therapy experience consisted of simply getting to and from each appointment. Next, I had to learn to walk again. I was taught how to lift things correctly, with the hope that I might someday be able to lift my daughter into her car seat. Picking things up from the floor was an advanced move that took lots of time and practice. At home, if something fell, it stayed there until I could beg a family member to pick it up.

Therapy started with simple steps. Pointing and flexing my toes, walking to and from my car, then farther. Walking a few houses down the street was a huge success. Sometimes a week would pass between these steps, but each brought more confidence.

These were challenging times. My husband began going to work late in order to take our younger daughter to preschool. I was grateful he could take her, because I was unable to walk up the stairs to the entrance to her school. At pickup, I needed to call for someone to walk her to my car.

It would take me thirty minutes to get out of bed every morning. The alarm would sound. I would yell out my older daughter's name from bed, and she would run in. After a restless night, I could usually convince her to lie in bed with me so mommy could sleep just a little while longer.

Next, I convinced myself to roll over, sit up, and finally stand. Still bent at the waist, I would slowly rise and gather energy to move. Taking it slowly, I would walk to the restroom and kitchen, holding onto every piece of furniture and all of the walls along the way. I would think, "If I can only get her to school, then I can come home and lie back down." My daughter made her own breakfast most mornings. Her lunch was pre-made by her father. Every day he called to make sure we were out of bed. It was all I could do to get dressed and out the door.

Each step forward is a step in the right direction. Never give up hope. Ever.

Yelling became a form of communication. I would yell from my room to say hello or ask for help as family arrived home. When one of the girls did something wrong, I yelled at her, because I wasn't able to pick her up and physically put her in time out. I yelled for water, food, everything. I felt much anger and resentment, and so sorry for myself. The physical pain increased as each day went on, so evenings were especially challenging. I needed more than just physical help.

That spring, my family had a special trip planned to Mexico. It had only been a few months since my diagnosis, but I really wanted to go. I used the trip to give me motivation. With the positive pressure to keep up with my exercises and the promise of help from my family, my doctors let me go.

I believed being away from home would take my troubles away. Magically, everything would be better in the sunshine and warmth. That turned out not to be true. I covered up my feelings every day. I weighed well over 200 pounds and should have been thinking of my health. Instead, I covered my pain and sadness with sugar, vodka, and comfort food.

During that trip, my husband and I had an opportunity to trade babysitting with friends, so we went on a date. None of my clothes fit, and I felt unhappy and self-conscious, but got dressed anyway, and we took a taxi ride to a nearby city. The pain from driving on the bumpy dirt roads was painful. We arrived in a small town with a beautiful beach and decided to take a walk before dinner.

As the sun set, I held my husband's hand. The beach was gorgeous, but I was crying. I was in so much pain, and had been trying to cover it up for what was supposed to be our romantic date. I gave in and asked my husband to take me home. I can't even remember if we ate dinner or not. I do, however, have a photo from that night: it is my "before" photo on the back of this book. I felt all alone, disgusted with my personal appearance, and sad. I had lost myself.

It was time for me to become the person I knew was waiting quietly inside me.

When we returned from our trip, I thought about the many things I wasn't able to enjoy. At my next physical therapy appointment, I watched another patient who seemed to be perfectly fine, like she didn't even belong in therapy. First came thoughts of anger and resentment toward her. Why was she making those of us who were recovering feel worse about where we were?

But then, something clicked inside me and I had a moment of clarity. I suddenly began to feel hope and inspiration that I, too, could recover and move like her.

What if I could get better? What if I didn't have to feel this way forever?

"Only in the darkness can you see the stars."
~Martin Luther King Jr.

I needed to change, if not for me, then for my family. My "why" became very apparent: I couldn't continue hurting the ones I loved. My older daughter was afraid to get near me for fear I would yell at her. I couldn't pick up my younger daughter to hug her, and often fell asleep while playing with her. Not knowing how else to help, my husband busied himself each night with housework and taking care of our beautiful girls. I wasn't even able to hug him due to the pain.

I was tired of lying on the couch, feeling sad and unworthy of love or hope. I needed to change for my family. They deserved a mother who could be present and a wife who could be loved.

Become inspired.

With new conviction and confidence, I set myself a simple goal: to walk our beautiful older daughter to school. She was in first grade at an elementary school four blocks from our home. Every morning, I would drive her to school, but many days, she didn't want a ride. Since I couldn't walk that far, I had to drive alongside her while she ran or walked on the sidewalk.

I was determined to walk her all the way to school, and my determination inspired me. I wanted to be an active mother again, not just watching my daughters' lives go by.

As I began to feel better, I would park near the school and attempt to walk with my daughter to the playground where her class lined up, but I was embarrassed and didn't want anyone to see me unable to walk well. Still, I stuck with it and used my daughter's desire and hope to inspire me, and I myself was hopeful. I practiced walking a block at a time. Each week, I walked a bit more.

When I finally believed I was ready to walk the entire four blocks, I got up early one morning to give my body time to warm up. I usually wore slip-on shoes, since I could hardly reach my feet. But that morning, I was able to tie my tennis shoes, with a little help from my daughter.

Believe in possibility.

We walked out the door of our house, her hand in mine. She began to skip, and I had to call her back to slow down. I took a deep breath and used her excitement to inspire me. We made it all the way to the playground! Less than half a mile in 15 minutes was a success! I watched her walk into school with a smile, and I shed tears of joy.

There was one problem: I wasn't sure I could get home, and was too embarrassed to ask for help. I leaned against the school fence for some time, then made it across the street to a bench. I had four blocks to go, and one of them was uphill. This was going to take some serious strength and mental focus.

I began to walk slowly, reminding myself with every step how far I had already come. I knew it was possible for me to do it. I kept my eyes forward and took each step with a deep breath. I approached the hill and shuffled up, holding a fence along the way. Reaching home, I had tears running down my face. I had walked my daughter to school. It was a great day!

My work was not done, however. Just six months after my diagnosis, I met a friend who introduced me to a community called Transformation.com by Bill Phillips. I used the Transformation.com exercises, along with accountability and support, to become lighter both physically and mentally. I took my health back, and used that momentum to carry me forward to greater goals. I believed that anything was possible and used that hope to become strong. And it all started with small goals accomplished.

Inspiration comes in many forms.

When I first began to walk, it took so much strength. In time, I became motivated to see how far I could go. The walking seemed to help my spine. Free movement, with arms swinging, started to feel good.

Inspired by my daughter, who was doing a children's marathon over the course of several weeks, I signed up to walk a half-marathon. I questioned if I could actually complete it, but chose to train anyway.

When I finally completed those 13.1 miles, I became very emotional. Raising money for autism research, a cause I care deeply about, gave me motivation to push through the tough times. I walked farther than I had ever walked. It wasn't easy, but it was simple: put one foot in front of the other, lean forward, and repeat.

Then, one day, I longed to move faster.

Runners are crazy; that is what I used to tell myself. But during a walk, I jogged a half block. Surprised I felt no pain, I walked a bit and jogged again. All good. I felt like I was flying.

"If you don't go after what you want, you'll never have it. If you don't ask, the answer is always no. If you don't step forward, you're always in the same place."
~Nora Roberts

After my history, asking a doctor for permission to begin running was going to be interesting. I remember his words exactly: "It sounds like I can't convince you not to, but if you run, it needs to be a smooth gallop, not a trot." I got the green light for an occasional jog to the corner. I felt alive and secretly ran farther than I was given permission to.

Running had never come easy to me. Yes, I ran a year of track in high school, but I hid every time we had to do more than a mile warm-up. The only other running I had done was during one summer in my early thirties, when my spine was strong and I completed 8k and 10k fun runs. My friend and I were the last to finish the 10k, but we finished.

Running is and will always be a challenge for me. Even at the level that I currently race, it is tough. I was the last female over forty to finish the first run leg of Duathlon Nationals last year, but I didn't let that stop me. I know how to change my shoes so I can transition quickly onto my bike and back into my run shoes for the second run. I usually pass several people on my bike ride while others are fussing with their gear.

Don't let one setback keep you from great things.

I had started endurance racing against all odds. Resistance seemed to come at every turn. While running, it was always very hard to breathe. After finding that I had a jogging heart rate of over 200 beats per minute, I saw a heart specialist and a pulmonary specialist and had several medical tests done. An EKG, echocardiogram, pulmonary lung function test, and several breathing tests later, I was diagnosed with athletic-induced asthma. I also learned I was allergic to dust and most trees—not great for a year-round runner who runs mainly outside on a forested trail in the city. I had thought it was challenging for everyone to breathe while running. No, it is not.

The medical tests all screamed: "You should NOT be an athlete for a living." Instead, I was prescribed inhalers, allergy medication, and iron supplements, and chose to face the challenge head on. I don't let my lungs define me. Instead I believe what is possible and rely on my other strengths.

Despite the many challenges I face, I have come to really enjoy exercising. I never thought that I could feel this way. Not only am I strengthening my heart and lungs, but I gain tremendous inner strength and confidence through exercise. During many workouts, I feel a profound sense of calm and meditation. This didn't happen overnight, but the more I gave into the rhythmic pattern of my heartbeat, footsteps, and breathing, the more I found peace.

Whatever you choose for exercise, I know you, too, can find peace. Be patient.

Although I had already achieved many goals, I desired to work on other challenges in my life. When I completed one goal, I quickly set another. Sometimes I set one prior to achieving the last one. I was constantly looking ahead—while still being present in my life.

Feeling "okay" and "just existing" were not options for me. Originally, that had been all I dreamed of. Now I wanted more, and I knew that it was possible. I could see it in my dreams and visualize it when I walked.

I knew that I needed to spend time repairing relationships with my husband, daughters, and friends. I needed to forgive myself and move past the resentment I held onto. While I was able to go back to work at a retail shop, I didn't feel appreciated there, so I looked for a place where I could thrive.

I wanted to feel the passion that I had felt for so many years. My life felt like a puzzle, all the pieces dropped and scattered on the floor. Hoping none were missing, I desperately tried to pick them up and begin the process of putting them back together, one section at time.

It is possible to find yourself again. I did.

At my first triathlon there was a sign that read, "I tri because I can!" After seeing it, I cried for the last mile. I was there because I *could,* when for so long, I truly couldn't. Finishing, I felt strong, happy, and confident. What an amazing feeling it is to be using your body. No one could take that away from me. It didn't matter how long it took me to finish, that I barely made it through the swim, or what I looked like when I did; I was active and fully participating in my life. I proved to myself and others that life can't be taken for granted.

Seize the day.

Life isn't about what we can't do, but rather what we CAN. For a few years I had a teammate who raced triathlons with only one arm. He swam faster than me, put on his own shoes and helmet quickly, and biked faster than me, too. When I get to feeling sorry for myself, I just remember that so many others have far greater challenges than I.

Do what you can to move forward and continue your climb.

Baby steps are still steps that move you forward in the direction of your dreams. My original goal of wanting to feel strong wasn't a physical goal, although that would have been nice. It was to feel worthwhile, able to make it through my day without crying or feeling like I was letting myself or someone else down.

Today, I choose to spend quality time with my family. I exercise six days a week and fuel my body with colorful and great tasting foods. I look for possibility in every situation and continue to learn and grow.

I am selfish and take time just for me every week. My family would rather have me away for a few hours, and then fully present afterward, than with them and distant, in pain, sad, or depressed. Self-care is of the utmost importance. If we choose not to take care of ourselves first, we won't have the energy or presence for those we love.

My spine will never be the same as it was when I was a child. I will always have to maintain an active life to keep my core and back

---

strong. But it is worth every ounce of sweat to continue living an active and pain-free life.

Not knowing if, or when, I will relapse, I remain in gratitude for all I am able to do each day. I prepare by staying strong mentally and physically. I take nothing for granted and continue to live a life where I can inspire others to live their best.

There is a light at the end of every tunnel, no matter how long it takes to find it.

I remember the first day that I didn't have to brace myself before my girls could run up and hug me.

I remember the day that I played with my girls at the park, not just watching them play alone.

I remember the day that I didn't cringe from pain when my husband lay next to me in bed.

I remember the day I gave my then-six-year-old her first piggyback ride.

I remember the little things that I used to take for granted, which now mean everything to me, and even more to my family.

I remember the day I CHOSE to take my life back and become *Mary* again.

My autographed photo is now in my spine specialist's office next to the other athletes he has helped. Be inspired by the little and big things, and believe that they are in your reach. I never imagined seeing my photo in that office back when I was suffering, in pain, and hardly able to walk. But anything is possible. There *is* hope.

You can become anything you imagine.

Acknowledge Where You Are

"Start where you are. Use what you have.
Do what you can." ~Arthur Ashe

First, take inventory of where you are now. You cannot get anywhere without knowing where you are starting from. This is where it all begins.

When you don't feel great about yourself, taking the time to look at yourself might not seem like the way you want to spend a free afternoon. I get it. But that is exactly what you have to do.

We often believe that if we ignore something we don't like, it will go away. In many cases this isn't because we don't care; it is more that we allowed other things to become more important in our lives. Priorities change, time passes, and all of a sudden we look up and see that we are not where we want to be.

The good news is that we looked up!

If we choose not to see where we are, we continue to be in denial about things that are not working in our lives. It could be our career, a relationship, health, spirituality, nutrition, or pieces of all of the above.

When I had two young children, I began to ignore my finances. Before that time, I could have told you at any given moment exactly how much money I had. I paid cash for everything, worked to pay off school as I went, and felt good about my financial situation. I had a good relationship with money. The busier I got, however, the less I thought about my finances. Not that it wasn't important, because it was, but I made other things more important.

I told myself that even if I didn't know how much we spent each month, it would all work out. My husband and I were careful with our money and not extravagant. By not paying attention, however, we spent more than we made. After taking a closer look, we became fully aware of our finances. We asked for help, held ourselves accountable, and did what we needed to do to make positive changes. We're now on track for a great retirement, with a budget and lifestyle we feel good about.

For some reason, it isn't ignoring the problem that causes us distress, but dwelling on it.

Do you feel resentment toward others who are thinner than you, who run better than you, or who are happily married? Do you resent someone who has a job you dream of, who travels, or who is happy? Do you envy someone who has children or does things you only dream of?

If not, then you are way further along in your journey to creating your best life than I was. But if so, you are not alone. I felt all of these things and more for over a decade. Even so, I was still closer than I ever imagined to becoming the person I was meant to be—to becoming my best self.

A few years ago I was sad, depressed, overweight, and resentful toward anyone who was healthy. Finances were tough. I felt tired all the time, in need of a hug, and distant—and I yelled a lot. I was impatient and in constant physical pain. I brought everyone around me down in order to feel better about myself.

Now I am living a wonderful life filled with joy, gratitude, possibility, happiness, health, and positive energy. I have a career that I enjoy. I am truly ALIVE. Did it happen overnight? No. But it did happen, and I know it can for you, too. So let's get started!

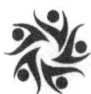

Stating the Facts

"The acceptance of responsibility

Is not the acceptance of a burden

But the multiplication of opportunity."

~Sri Chinmoy

When thinking about your current state, it is best to keep your thoughts judgment-free. This will not be easy. We are emotional beings who take everything personally. I know I did. Moreover, I did not like anyone telling me what to do, how to do it, or how to change. Just remember that this is challenging but doable. Breathe.

State the facts. You are what you are, and it won't help move you forward if you choose to be hard on yourself. So find a quiet place to sit, close your eyes, and take ten slow and deep breaths through your nose. Think about who and where you are in your life today. Do you feel good? Sad? Challenged? Unfulfilled? Happy? Encouraged? Where do you feel "full" and where do you feel "lacking"?

Soon you will learn about Primary and Secondary Foods™. When you think about each of these areas of your life, you might find that one or two are not where you would like them to be. If so, I will invite you to ask yourself, "What would I like to be different?"

Remember to be good to yourself and judgment-free.

For many of us, there was a certain point in our life when we just let a piece of us go. We often reminisce about what it was like "in the good old days" or dream of a different future. We can't go back, and the future is uncertain, but what we do have is the here and now. So take action today to start living the future you dream about for your tomorrow.

Important Life Elements

"You only live once, but if you do it right,
once is enough." ~Mae West

There are four primary areas of our lives:

- Relationships
- Physical activity
- Career
- Spirituality

These four areas make up our **Primary Food**™ ². Nutrition and "real" food is actually considered **Secondary Food**™ ². Let me explain.

Primary Food is so important. When your four Primary Foods are in alignment, balanced, and working together, this deeper form of nutrition is in alignment. But when even one of these areas is lacking, we need to focus on changing it to create more cohesion in our lives. Let's talk about these very important elements that make up life.

RELATIONSHIPS

Our relationships with family, friends, partners, children, and co-workers shape our lives. Those we choose to surround ourselves with will encourage, inspire, love, and grow old with us. They will also share joy, happiness, sadness, and despair with us.

"If conversation was the lyrics, laughter was the music, making time spent together a melody that could be replayed over and over without getting stale." ~Nicholas Sparks

Do you feel supported by your family? Do you have a partner or someone you can trust to call at any hour of the day or night to share your most exciting wins or most challenging life moments? It is very important to have someone in your life whom you can depend on. It's also great if, in return, they can also depend on you.

With the digital world as it is, we don't have to step a foot out the door, or even pick up the phone, in order to connect. But humans—and all mammals—are physical creatures. We also need human touch, hugs, and pats on the back. Even a simple smile can generate such positivity in our day. Do you spend time with friends physically and in person, or just via phone and Internet?

When we talk about people we share our lives with, this also includes the people we work with each day. Do your co-workers bring you good energy and joy, or are they hard on you? Do they make you feel less than you are? Would you feel comfortable going to lunch or taking a break with them, or would you rather eat alone than spend time with them?

"Never lose sight of the fact that the most important yardstick of your success will be how you treat other people—your family, friends, and coworkers, and even strangers you meet along the way." ~Barbara Bush

There are certain people in your life whose appearance makes you feel instantly better because they draw you toward them with their wonderful energy. Who do you know that brings you that kind of joy and energy, just by their presence? Wouldn't it be great if you could spend more time with them? How could you make that happen?

PHYSICAL EXERCISE

Movement of any kind that gets our heart pumping while keeping our muscles and bones strong is wonderful for our bodies. Exercise gives us mental clarity and helps us sleep and recover faster. Movement can be anything from housework, to yard work, to a physical career, to daily or weekly workouts in a gym.

Take a look at your average week. What type of exercise do you do? How long do you exercise within each workout time? No matter what type of movement you do, write it down. Parking farther away at the grocery store counts! If you enjoy a career that is very physical, you might not need as much additional movement in order to get healthy heart exercise throughout your work week.

Or maybe you are the type of person who gets your movement in when you are preparing for and getting to work, or doing housework. Are you also taking additional time during the week to lift weights, take a walk, swim, enjoy a yoga class, run, ski, cycle, dance, or something else you enjoy?

"My grandmother started walking five miles a day when she was sixty. She's ninety-seven now, and we don't know where the heck she is." ~Ellen DeGeneres

Are you someone who likes to exercise at home, outside, or in a gym? When I first began an exercise program again, I was put off by going into a gym full of fit people. But what I soon noticed is that everyone is there for the same reason: to stay or become healthy.

Other people, myself included, enjoy exercising outside. Anyone with a pair of sneakers can head outside, anytime and most anywhere, to get their heart pumping. When I was able, walking was my movement of choice. Not only was I getting fresh air, increased health, and movement to my spine, I often got what I like to call a "free facial." When you live in Seattle, misty or rainy mornings are great for your skin.

"An early morning walk is a blessing
for the whole day." ~Henry David Thoreau

Do you exercise with friends, family, or on your own? One of the things I enjoy about running or cycling is that I can do it alone. It is my time to reconnect to nature, think through my day, let it all go, and enjoy hearing the sounds of my footsteps and heartbeat. Even though most of my exercise is done alone, there is something undeniable about exercising with another.

I have fond memories of a few years' worth of regular early morning walks with a good friend. We shared our thoughts, dreams, and hopes while walking. We consoled one another and laughed a bit, too. And group exercise classes bring me energy for days. I love the positive pressure and motivation I receive from others with similar health goals. Yes, we are there for our own health, but when we are all suffering together, there is a sense of camaraderie that motivates me to work harder and not give up.

What type of exercise would you choose to do if you could create more time and find a way to fit it into your current schedule? When we make priorities for our health, and put ourselves on our own calendar, we *can* manage to fit in our workouts. It can take some creativity, but it is worth it. Most people experience greater mental clarity and an ability to complete work more quickly throughout their day after a morning workout. I know that I also sleep better when I have exercised in any given day. Sleep is critical for overall health, as that is the time when our bodies are recovering from our day and growing, and cells are healing us from the inside.

CAREER

No matter what you have chosen to do for work in your life, you should enjoy it. Yes, there will always be times when a part of our everyday duties includes something that we don't particularly care for, but all in all, we should feel good about what we accomplish each day. Whether you are a stay-at-home parent, student, artist, volunteer, office worker, or medical professional—or any other type of professional—you get to choose how you spend your days.

"The crowning fortune of a man is to be born to some pursuit which finds him employment and happiness, whether it be to make baskets, or broadswords, or canals, or statues, or songs." ~Ralph Waldo Emerson

Let's talk about your career. What have you chosen to do for a living? Is it a job that you can't wait to get up in the morning for, because it brings you such energy and life? Does your career also bring you the funds that you need to live?

Many people feel obligated to continue in a career they don't enjoy in order to feed family or pay the bills. Sometimes this can't be helped, but then it is important to look for a hobby that brings pure joy and passion. Those who use their passion to create a job that becomes a fulfilling career reach even greater daily joy.

"I've learned that making a 'living' is not the same thing as 'making a life.'" ~Maya Angelou

Ask yourself, are you passionate about what you do such that you can hardly believe you are getting paid to enjoy it? Take some time to think about a career or job that you have always dreamed of doing but held yourself back from due to lack of education, age, finances, or geography. What if none of these things were obstacles? What would you choose then?

SPIRITUALITY

No matter what you believe in or how you bring it into your life, believing in something greater than yourself can clear your mind, allow you to become more present in your day, and bring you a greater sense of inclusion in this world.

Scheduling time each week for quiet is rarely done. We are trying so hard to pack as much into our days as possible that we forget to look up or take a breath. And for some, quiet can be scary. If you have always lived a life of chaos, that is all you know. When we force ourselves to spend time alone or in a state of calm, it can take some time before our body allows us to truly settle down and begin to listen to our heart.

> *"A quiet conscience makes one strong!"*
> *~Anne Frank, The Diary of a Young Girl*

When we choose to quiet our mind, we invite an inner peace that we so need. Do you regularly participate in yoga, meditation, walking after dinner, or other activities that slow you down and bring you back into the present?

For some, spirituality can mean religion, or the belief that there is a power greater than ourselves. Do you attend church or another organized religious or spiritual service with family or friends? If so, this can be a time to stop thinking about what is troubling you. Instead, use the time to get closer to your inner thoughts and also grow closer to your family, friends, and community of like-minded individuals—all with the purpose of celebrating the good and living your best life.

> "The greatest disease in the West today is not TB or leprosy; it is being unwanted, unloved, and uncared for. We can cure physical diseases with medicine, but the only cure for loneliness, despair, and hopelessness is love. There are many in the world who are dying for a piece of bread but there are many more dying for a little love. The poverty in the West is a different kind of poverty—it is not only a poverty of loneliness but also of spirituality. There's a hunger for love, as there is a hunger for God."
> ~Mother Teresa, A Simple Path: Mother Teresa

If you could make more time to incorporate quiet and reflection into your life, how would you choose to spend it? How could it take your life to the next level, bringing you a greater feeling of gratitude and peace? I know that when I allow my mind to sit still, after all the chaos passes by, I come to a state of inner peace, calm, and love that I need to live my best each day.

NUTRITION

Nutrition is another area of our lives that we need to pay attention to. How we choose to feed ourselves each day dictates how we feel and move through life. We often use food for more than just fueling our bodies, so we need to really think about why we are eating what we eat. This is why nutrition is considered "Secondary Food."

For most of us, nutrition suffers when it is used to alter our emotional state when one or more Primary Foods are out of balance. We think that it can help us, but eating emotionally only seems to work for a short time and is quickly followed by regret, guilt, and self-hate. Are you eating for life, eating for emotions you wish you were feeling, or eating to celebrate when something goes your way? Emotions that lead us to eat can be either challenging or positive, but the outcome is still the same when we over-indulge in foods we enjoy, comfort foods from our childhood, or foods we think we deserve but which don't yield any true nutritional value.

> *"Let food be thy medicine and medicine*
> *be thy food." ~Hippocrates*

Another reason our nutrition can suffer is pure boredom. Ever sit in front of a television or computer and find that an entire bag of chips has been devoured, when you only planned on eating a few? If so, you might be someone who eats when bored.

Do you drink, smoke, or add other things to your body that are unhealthy? I wouldn't consider these things "nutrition" in the way I do fruits, vegetables, minerals, fat, protein, and carbohydrates, but they are something humans use to redirect emotions, just like food. Think about the reasons why you choose to put these things into your body.

Food = fuel. The true motivation for our nutrition should be to gain fuel. We need hydration and food in order to give our bodies energy; without it we would perish. With loving preparation, we can give our food new meaning. What percent of your meals are home-cooked by you or a partner or family member? Do the other foods you eat come from restaurants or pre-prepared food establishments for on-the-go eating?

"I was 32 when I started cooking;
up until then, I just ate."

"You don't have to cook fancy or
complicated masterpieces—just good
food from fresh ingredients."

~Julia Child

When we take the time to prepare our own food, not only do we know all the ingredients and where they came from, we also have taken the time to prepare it in a caring way that can bring us even greater health. What would your meals and preparation time look like if you had all the time in the world to explore new options? Take the time to find recipes, learn from friends, ask co-workers, or take a cooking class. Get to know the foods you eat, where they come from, and how they are grown, and put some love into making them. Start simple, and then get more creative.

WHAT DEFINES YOU?

"When I let go of what I am,
I become what I might be."
~Lao Tzu

When we think of what defines us, the quick answer is on the surface: daughter, father, mother, husband, sister, friend, uncle, co-worker, teacher. However, what I am asking you to look for is much deeper than a job or relationship title... or is it?

For years I was a dancer, the daughter of two teachers, "number five" (sibling order out of six), business student, partner, and wife. Then life happened. My spine was injured, and suddenly I went from being seen as a healthy dancer and daughter to being seen as "one who is injured."

No matter what I was doing, people would come to my rescue to help me carry things. Of course I was grateful for the support and help while recovering, but years later, when my spine was healed and I no longer needed help, I was still perceived as the injured one with a bad back.

I ran half-marathons, and still no one let me carry my own luggage or groceries. Friends wanted to hold onto the person that I used to be and didn't see the strong woman I had become. I knew I was stronger than most of them, but they continued to see me as weak, so it made me believe it, too. Was I ready to really live? Maybe not, if my family and friends didn't believe it.

Don't let what currently defines you hold you back from your dreams. The things that define us can be from childhood, school years, an injury, accident, or simply what we look like. They can be related to not just who we are on the outside, but on the inside as well.

We not only let others in our life define who we are, but we give ourselves labels that can define us for years. Most of us would never let other people talk to us the way we talk to ourselves. You might call yourself fat, tired, old, stressed, ugly, lazy, or poor. But would you turn around and tell someone close to you that they were any one of these things in the same unkind manner you tell it to yourself? Most would not. So stop and take action. Take pride in who you are by choosing to create change and stand up for yourself.

Others' Thoughts Make Me Believe It Is So

"Never be bullied into silence. Never allow yourself to be made a victim. Accept no one's definition of your life; define yourself." ~Harvey Fierstein

Many things can define us: things that happened in our past, who we are in the present, the way others perceive us to be. Sometimes we give people permission to feel the way they do about us by our own words or actions. For instance, many of us grew up being called "the big guy" or "the nerdy girl" because of the way we looked or acted. But those words can stick with us for years and hurt our feelings.

For some reason, society deems it okay to create nicknames for people without asking for their permission. Some of these names stick and become lasting identity. How can we ask all of our family and friends to stop calling us something if they have been calling us that for years?

And even if you spend years trying to become someone different, there will always be those who, for selfish reasons, want to hang on to who you have always been to them. Often, it is because those people see themselves standing still and don't like that you are moving forward. After all, misery loves company, right? No one wants to feel left behind in a challenging, changing world.

When friends become resentful about the changes you are making, it can be challenging. You do not want to hurt feelings, but at the same time, you feel a strong desire to take care of yourself... and you should. You cannot hold onto labels that others give you in order to make them feel better.

Even after we make great changes in our own lives, there will still be times when our friends believe we should go back to our old ways. You have a choice. To appease others, you could spend time at locations or with people who don't have your best interests in mind "for the night," taking the risk of slipping away from your goal. Or, you could offer other suggestions for things to do, and share why you feel this way. By choosing the best for your own life you might inspire others to make changes in their lives, too. Become the person you were meant to be and live your best life. Some of the people who won't understand your changes initially will later stand in line to ask for advice. They won't choose differently because of your words, but instead because of your actions and choices in life.

Growing Up

"My father gave me the greatest gift anyone could give another person, he believed in me." ~Jim Valvano

The location, religion, sibling order, and era you grew up in can define you. Do you have an older sibling or parent with an interesting job or family business that you feel obligated to continue for another generation? Does your religion dictate what type of careers a woman or man should do, or whom you should marry?

There can be so much pressure to do as your parents or older siblings have done. We put some of that pressure on ourselves, but most comes from those around us. We are taught at an early age to listen to what others think of us and are encouraged to fulfill those expectations.

What we aren't always taught is that each of us is unique and should be celebrated as such.

We all have hopes, dreams, goals, and a vision of what will bring us passion, love, or hope. We need to realize our own destiny, not that of others. Unfortunately, this destiny isn't always what those around us believe it should be. Children of lawyers or doctors often become lawyers and doctors. But is that what you truly want for yourself, or are you doing it for someone else?

If your parents didn't go to college, you might not have the resources to go—or even be inspired to do so—unless someone provides encouragement. There is no shortage of examples where your past can define your present. It is your challenge to choose which things you want to define you. You get to take the good and change those things you don't care for. The possibilities are truly endless.

I take pride in being defined as the following things from my past: I am the daughter of two schoolteachers who have been married for over fifty years, the fifth of six children, a Girl Scout, and a volunteer. I like being known as a college graduate who paid her own way through school, a drummer since age ten, a dancer, and one who loves both music and math.

What do you like being defined by from your past?

For a long while, I lost my way and didn't feel healthy or strong. I was injured and let that define every part of me. My lack of health consumed me, and I used it as an excuse for many things. Several years ago, I chose to let that go, and now I define myself as the following.

I AM... Mary! Wife, Mother, Sister, Daughter, Aunt,

Friend, Athlete, Artist, Speaker, Author, Student of

Life, Inspiration for All... Caring, Passionate, Loving,

Compassionate, Grateful. I AM HEALTHY and

STRONG to live the life I know I can!

I remember the day that I added "Athlete" to the above statement. It was not the day I completed my first race or could run three miles. It was the day I chose to start moving again and not let my injuries keep me from feeling alive.

What would you like to be defined by now and in your future?

Take some time to think about your "I AM..." statement. Make it define all of the amazing things about who you are today and who you WILL be in the future.

What Song Is Playing in Your Head?

*"When I let go of what I am, I become
what I might be." ~Lao Tzu*

Each of us has a song. It might be the Rolling Stones, Motown, the Beatles, Beethoven, or Barry White. But it is ours. Whether we like it or not, we listen to it all too often. We hum it, sing it, hear it, believe it, and often become it.

From when we were very young, we were fed statements like "you aren't good enough," "you're the smart kid," or "you're just a jock." As a child, we trusted those around us and allowed these "songs" to record in our heads and play day after day... and we still believe them. They don't always make sense, but we go on living them out. Why? Because they are what we know.

You don't have to be a child to receive these messages; friends, spouses, employers, and society can give them to you, too. Some of us have several playing in our heads at once. Conflicting messages make it challenging for us to choose which to listen to. If a parent says "You won't amount to anything" and a favorite teacher says "You are capable of great things; don't ever let anyone tell you differently," you have a challenge. Whom do you believe? The person who is raising you and feeding you, or the person who you trust to teach you?

The voice you hear the most will be the one that plays most often in the shuffle that is your mind.

Ah, the shuffle button. Don't you wish you could switch it off? If we knew which negative song was coming up next, we could at least prepare ourselves with beautiful and inspirational thoughts to combat it. Instead, songs come at us when we least expect them, and unfortunately, the songs of hope do not generally come when we are sad and need them; they usually come when we are already happy. It just works that way. More often than not, we attract the types of thoughts that we are already feeling in the moment, not the ones we truly need. The exciting part is, we do have a choice. We get to choose to listen to those songs... or not. Is it easy to replace them with new songs? No. But when you want great change in your life that will redefine you, *you must change the songs*. Or, I should say, you GET to change them.

This is the great part. When we know what we want to become, we give ourselves new songs to listen to—or mantras, based on our ideals—which help us to become the person we know we can be.

How Is It Helping Me to Stay the Same?

"When I look back over my life it's almost as if there was a plan laid out for me—from the little girl who was so passionate about animals who longed to go to Africa and whose family couldn't afford to put her through college. Everyone laughed at my dreams. I was supposed to be a secretary in Bournemouth." ~Jane Goodall

We stay the same because it is easy and comfortable, or so we think. Not only does everyone already know who we are, we don't have to forge our way through resistance in order to make change. So why do it?

If you are okay living a life that is just "okay," and getting by day to day, then sure, keep on living as you are. However, I don't think you really are okay with the status quo, or you wouldn't be reading this book. I believe you want a better life; you want to make big changes, but just aren't sure how to go about doing it.

You have been through the "what ifs" and dreaming of "what could be." But have you really dug deep to think about how staying the same could affect the rest of your life?

"To live is the rarest thing in the world. Most people exist, that is all." ~Oscar Wilde

If you dream of having a partner to share your life with, but by the age of ninety haven't found one, what regrets will you have? If you dream of traveling to Europe and exploring ancient cities, but are now too fragile or injured to make the journey, will you look back on your younger years with sadness?

We think that staying the same is easy. However, if we truly think about it, it's not as easy as we think. Change is inherent. The world keeps turning, the rivers keep flowing whether or not we choose to change. If we do not move forward, then we choose nothing. There is no standing still. To remain the same, we must actually move backward while the rest of the world moves forward at its own pace. You won't ever find the perfect time to make big changes in your life. So do it today.

"In Italy for thirty years under the Borgias they had warfare, terror, murder, and bloodshed, but they produced Michelangelo, Leonardo da Vinci, and the Renaissance. In Switzerland, they had brotherly love; they had five hundred years of democracy and peace, and what did that produce? The cuckoo clock." ~Orson Welles

Some of my clients, for instance, tell me it is too hard and expensive to eat healthy food all the time. I sometimes respond by asking them how much their medical bills were last year, or how much their bills might be if they choose to stay on their current path of unhealthy eating and end up developing a debilitating disease as a consequence.

Some say staying in the same unfulfilling career is fine. I ask them how they feel at the end of each day. Some tell me that they feel "okay" about their relationships. I then ask, "Wouldn't you like to feel incredible, unbelievable, and excited to go home to your partner?" Life is what we make of it.

Are you still convinced that staying the same is what you want for the rest of YOUR life?

We need to stop and think about the consequences of NOT achieving our goals. If the answer is a resounding "YES, I will regret not trying," then you have to go after your dreams and goals today. Stop waiting for the right time. There is no such thing. I was watching a television program on New Year's Eve and someone was asked how she felt about resolutions. She answered brilliantly, saying, "If you aren't willing to start making a change today, then it might not be worth starting at all." Not to say that being inspired by a new year isn't wonderful. But, we mustn't wait until a holiday—or next Monday—to begin. We just have to be brave and go for it, if it is important to us.

car·pe di·em noun \\'kär-pe-'dē-,em, -'dī-, -əm\\ Latin, literally, "pluck the day." First known use: 1817. The enjoyment of the pleasures of the moment without concern for the future.[3]

Carpe diem. Seize the day. Today is that day. If you pride yourself on living in the present, tomorrow will never come.

All it takes is you, a dream, and determination.

I opened a flower and gift store when I had a nine-month-old baby, and everyone around me thought I was crazy. I had dreamed of owning a store for years, but in fear, hadn't expressed it. Others didn't know that I needed to get out of the house for my sanity. Having a fulfilling career and happiness beyond family was important to me.

Being surrounded by things that I loved in my shop, including my new small child, gave me so much joy. While some women feel satisfied as stay-at-home mothers, sitting at home made me feel alone and helpless. I needed to go after my dreams, no matter how unreal they might seem.

I am grateful to have had a supportive husband who believed in me, which made things much easier. No matter what, I had to follow my heart. It wasn't easy, and I had to endure many challenges along the way, but I would have kicked myself had I not taken the risk to go after what I knew I needed.

Is it helping YOU to stay the same? I once chose to live on the sidelines of life because I thought it was easier for life to happen *to me* instead of choosing how I wanted my life to be. What I found is that it was much more challenging to try to stay the same in an ever-changing world than it was to forge through the thicket that I had allowed to grow around me. Then I saw a path of light coming through.

Set aside the emotions, breathe, and take a leap of faith. You will not regret it.

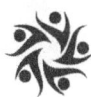

WHAT DO YOU LOVE?

*"Don't aim for success if you want it; just
do what you love and believe in, and it
will come naturally." ~David Frost*

What are things that make you come to life with exuberant joy, happiness, and excitement? These are the things you LOVE. Whether it is a person, place, or thing you love, being able to live in a state where you are reminded of what you love daily is important. Personally, when I was able to do that, I began to fully live in the present and feel alive.

*"If you do what you love, you'll never work
a day in your life." ~Marc Anthony*

When you combine love with gratitude, there is a sense of completeness that comes over whatever you are doing. In challenging times, it can be tough to visualize what that might feel like. I know because I chose to stay in that place for many years.

By finding those things that bring you pure joy, you are bringing things back into your life that you love. As you add more of those things, you crowd out the things that take energy away from you and bring you down.

Let me help you rediscover what YOU love.

I Have Passion

"Passion is one great force that unleashes creativity, because if you're passionate about something, then you're more willing to take risks." ~Yo-Yo Ma

When I think of the word *passion*, I think of something that lights me up, makes me smile, gives me hope, and brings the *possibility* back into my vocabulary as well. Think of some things that bring passion into your life. When you choose to add more of these things, the cost of having to make time for them no longer seems as daunting.

When we choose to engage in things that we love and are passionate about, we wake up with excitement for the day and seem to lose track of time. These things we love bring us energy and an enthusiasm about sharing with others so we don't collapse or run out of energy at the end of our day. Think of a time when you were doing an activity for a long stretch of time and became so lost with joy that you didn't even remember to stop and eat.

"Find something you're passionate about and keep tremendously interested in it." ~Julia Child

Take some time to think about what gives you energy and passion in your life. Think of things which are so enjoyable that they don't even qualify as real work—things you would do for free if you could. Too many of us continue to do the same type of work year after year, not even considering other things that might bring us much greater joy.

Think of something that you would cancel most anything for in order to get to do. Is there something that you would wake up much earlier than normal for? That thing is your passion. Think about how you could bring more of it into your life.

For me, there are certain activities that I smile to even think about doing. Likewise, certain people have a way of bringing me joy and making me come to life. What are some activities or people *you* spend time with that give you feel-good energy?

The good news is that, with passion in our lives, we tend to choose healthier lifestyles. We live full and promising lives and no longer use food to suppress negative emotions and fears.

Dream Big

"Return to your childhood's

Forgotten dreams.

You will be able to expedite

The fulfillment of your life's realities."
~Sri Chinmoy

Now that you know exactly what you are passionate about, you are ready to begin to dream. This is the fun part. Recall things from your childhood, lost dreams that you let go of for others, or interests and passions that truly resonate with you. What if you went after these now, as an adult?

Dreams are amazing and can lead us to becoming who we were truly meant to be.

When I was a child, I wanted to become an art teacher when I grew up. Although that didn't happen, it turns out that I do love to teach, and I love art. In some way, the "art teacher" idea stayed with me into adulthood. But at a certain point, I was ready to take a closer look at what could help me live up to my true calling in life.

When you were a child, what did *you* dream of doing? Are there things from your past that you gave up in order to make more time for other things, believing you didn't have room for both?

We often believe there isn't enough time in our day to engage in the things we are passionate about and still spend time with people we love. I myself experienced this when I had children: my husband and I had always enjoyed going to art galleries and movies together, but we stopped doing these things when the kids were born. And before we got married, he enjoyed playing soccer. But children and marriage made us believe we had to choose between the things we enjoyed and spending quality time together as a family.

Of course, making sacrifices for more family time is not a bad thing, but if giving up the things you love altogether takes away some of the happiness and joy in your life, that isn't good. After all, we can't pass on our joy to our children if we don't have any to give.

If you were to be given millions of dollars, tax-free, and never had to work for money again, what would you do with your newly gained time?

> "Sometimes I've believed as many as six impossible things before breakfast." ~Lewis Carroll

Do you remember a time when you were young and could spend time dreaming under a tree, reading an inspiring book, or hearing a great song? In those moments, you allowed your mind to wander to the realm of possibility. We can do that as adults, too. We sometimes need to work a bit harder to get there mentally, but we can do it if we believe we can. When you daydream as an adult, what do you imagine yourself doing? Where do you live, what do you do for fun?

Take some time to dream.

Create Meaning In Your Life

> *"Find out who you are and be that person. That's what your soul was put on this earth to be. Find that truth, live that truth, and everything else will come." ~Ellen DeGeneres*

When you leave this earth, the eulogist won't ask your family to describe how many hours you spent working or how you returned all of your emails within twenty-four hours. No one will care that your home was kept immaculately clean, or even that you had the most beautiful clothing or the coolest cars.

Instead, they will remember how much you loved your family and often spent quality time with them. Likely, they will share what you accomplished in your life that helped others, how you gave back in service, and any other things that brought joy, happiness, or love to others.

Of course, it's a somewhat dreary thought to consider what you will leave behind as a legacy when you die, but that is exactly what I think of when I want to create deep meaning in my life. How would your friends and family describe your current life to others?

We all have people that we know are a good example of what we would like to be. Think of someone you feel this way about. What qualities does he or she have that you admire? Whenever I see someone who carries with him a spectacular amount of love and joy for what he does or how he lives, I can not only see it in his eyes, but I can also feel it in his energy.

Can you recall a time when you felt that way about someone? Someone whose very entrance into a room gave you a good vibe, and you found yourself drawn to him? What if that person were actually you? Not because of your big wallet, or dashing looks, but because you chose life, love, and a compassionate way of living?

"The fullness of life

Lies in dreaming and manifesting

The impossible dreams." ~Sri Chinmoy

It is never too late to redefine who you are and what you stand for. Even if you have worked ten-hour days for years, it doesn't mean that you are stuck doing so forever. If you love what you do, and that work is important to you, great; if not, then it's time to make some changes now.

Or if a career change isn't possible, find a hobby that you love. There are other ways you can add value to your life. You could choose to give back by sharing what you know. You could spend more quality time with your family. Whatever that means to you, do it today.

Give yourself some time to think about the things that add meaning to your life and bring it value.

Some say life is short. I say life begins when you choose to start living.

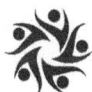

SMALL STEPS TURN INTO GIANT LEAPS

"The distance is nothing; it is only the first step that is difficult." ~Marie de Vichy-Chamrond, Marquise du Deffand, letter to Jean Le Rond d'Alembert, July 7, 1763

Taking the first step toward any goal or dream is never easy, but it can be done. Just breathe and dive in. The fear that we often feel, wondering what it will be like, is far worse than it ever can be. So what if you don't make it through day one? You get up and do it again the next day.

Nothing worthwhile is ever going to be easy. You knew that from the start. But the process can be simple. After setting intentions, knowing what you desire, and holding the "reasons why" close to your heart, you will succeed. You just have to make the first step, then lean forward so the second and third steps come a bit easier.

I want to share with you something that I wrote in my journal just six months after I decided to take my life back, and ten months after being diagnosed with severe spinal injuries.

I am so proud of the woman I was because she had the STRENGTH to seek out inspiration when she was so desperately in need.

She was in physical pain daily, depressed, and had no passion left in her life.

She had the COURAGE to literally JUMP headfirst into the challenge and try her best to eat well and begin an exercise program that she could do even with her physical limitations at the time.

She was CONFIDENT enough to continue when struggles arose... and they did.

She NEVER gave up HOPE, and continued even when she didn't think she could.

I COULDN'T BE MORE PROUD OF WHO I WAS... because I now know deep down inside that HER BEST QUALITIES NOW SHINE IN ME.

NEVER stop BELIEVING in YOURSELF.

Measurable Goals

"Goals are dreams with deadlines." ~Diana Scharf Hunt

I will never forget the day I chose to take my first step, and I celebrate it each year. You won't forget your "first steps" either.

When you are ready to start writing down your goals, you need to be specific about exactly what you want and how you are going to get it.

Setting goals is like using a good GPS system: you can program it to lead you "somewhere beautiful," but you won't get there without the specific details of where you would like to go. Without enough input, the navigation system might bring you to a neighborhood garden, but will it take you to a particular beach? Not unless you set the coordinates.

"If you aim at nothing, you will hit it every time." ~attributed to Zig Ziglar

There are a few types of goals that you need to consider. Long-term goals are just what they sound like. They are things that are grander than something you can achieve in a few weeks' time. I find long-term goals incredibly important to keep me on track and constantly moving forward.

Each year I choose one or two larger goals so that I know in what direction I am headed. There are always course corrections along the way, but I like to have some structure to my life. In the past, when I didn't do this, things did not turn out so great. For me, structure requires accountability, and with good accountability brings achievement.

Beginning something new can be daunting, so breaking your larger goals up into smaller ones will help you hold focus on reaching your long-term objectives. Short-term goals are often steps toward our long-term goals. Bigger goals are more easily achieved when we break them apart.

By checking smaller accomplishments off your list quickly, you will see progress on a weekly and monthly basis. This will bring wonderful forward momentum. Each time you successfully complete a small goal, you will receive a gift of confidence. With that, you are more likely to continue toward the completion of your much larger goals.

Life goals help define the way you live your life. These are broad goals. Keeping a list of these handy will give you a constant reminder of how you want, and choose, to live. Some call these types of goals *intentions*.

I'll talk a little bit more about each of these types of goals in the next few sections.

Long-Term Goals

"You must have long-range goals to keep you from being frustrated by short-range failures." ~Charles C. Noble

When you think of something that you long to achieve, how does it make you feel? If it makes you feel both excited and nervous at the same time, then you are likely on the right track. Remember to think beyond what you think is possible *now*. Long-term goals are usually something that you want to achieve in the next one to two years. Larger dreams come true only if given the time needed to achieve them.

When I first began my initial transformation from couch potato to endurance athlete, all I wanted was to feel strong inside and out. It didn't seem like that big of a deal at the time, but it was huge. As someone who had lost control of her life due to injury, sadness, and an identity crisis, I know all too well how having a seemingly simple goal can change one's life forever. I started simple and added larger goals as I went. Personally, having a long-term goal to work toward set me on a path of forward momentum that would eventually bring me to a much clearer, healthier, and active life. My goal was simple, but it brought me to a place where I could begin to truly live again.

> *"All our dreams can come true—if we have courage to pursue them."* ~Walt Disney

Take a moment to think about a goal or two that you truly want to achieve this year. These should be goals that you would regret not going after when you look back in five years.

Dream big, make it a bit uncomfortable to achieve. That is how you will rise to the occasion.

Short-Term Goals

> *"On this day all beginnings are created and all endings imagined."* ~Yuroz

When we truly commit to a well-thought-out goal, we set ourselves up for success. Whatever we choose to do with our 24 hours a day, we need to make sure it is important. We often spend so much time putting out small fires that we no longer have any time left in our days to engage in what actually gives us passion and energy for life.

"You miss 100 percent of the shots you don't take." ~Wayne Gretzky

Take a moment to think about the smaller goals that will enable you to achieve your long-term goals. These will keep you moving forward during the next few months. Just like your larger goals, without specific dates and ways to measure your short-term goals, there cannot be accountability.

This is where we get down to business. Create short-term goals that will keep you moving forward each and every day.

At the back of this book (and on my website at www.LiveAliveFit.com), there are Action Steps to help you organize and achieve your goals. Feel free to skip ahead now and start using them to set and keep your short- and long-term goals.

Life Goals and Intentions

"One half of knowing what you want is knowing what you must give up before you get it." ~Sidney Howard

When I think of lifetime goals and intentions, I think of how I want to live my life. I ask myself what purpose I want to give my days. It is important to be able to ask myself, at any moment, am I moving closer to or further away from my goals?

Below are a set of my personal life goals and intentions so that you can get an idea of what is possible. Use these to inspire your intentions for your own life.

Remember that your life goals and intentions will always be a working document. Please do not feel pressure to decide your entire future today. My list of goals and intentions has evolved many times since I first wrote them down years ago.

These life goals and intentions are something you will want to come back to from time to time—perhaps every six months or once a year. My own example is only intended to help give you overall direction along your newly created life path.

Mary's Personal Life Goals and Intentions:

- ❋ *To live the life I was intended to live and be the strongest and healthiest that I can be, inside and out, so that I can inspire others to live with passion and be their best people too.*

- ❋ *To be an example to my daughters and all young girls about what it is like to be a healthy woman who is loving, caring, giving, hopeful, and strong!*

- ❋ *To continue to learn, help others, and be an advocate for children and women.*

- ❋ *To set regular short- and long-term goals in order to continue to be strong inside and out, while also growing spiritually.*

- ❋ *To give back in any way I am able, share my artistic gifts, and inspire others to find their true passion in life.*

- ❋ *To be able to look back and know I lived a life full of love, passion, and faith... always giving more than I took.*

Give yourself some time to stop and think about how you hope to live your life. What do you want your legacy to be? What brings you joy and energy? With these things in mind, take the time to write down a few things that resonate with the way you want to live in order to always be your true self. These are not necessarily things that you are doing today, but ways you would ultimately like to live each day in order to be who you want to be. They will help you grow closer to the life that you were intended to live.

Making Time for Me

"Don't say you don't have enough time. You have exactly the same number of hours per day that were given to Helen Keller, Pasteur, Michelangelo, Mother Teresa, Leonardo da Vinci, Thomas Jefferson, and Albert Einstein." ~H. Jackson Brown, Jr.

When we think about starting something new in our lives, we sometimes aren't sure how we are going to fit it all into our days. The first step to making it work is to ask yourself *what is most important*.

If you are not happy now, it might be worth taking a closer look at how you spend your time. What you do each day is a mirror of your life's priorities. What do you spend the most time doing outside of work and family time? If you placed an order of importance in your life, would the hours you spend each week doing those things match your list in order of priority?

Life gets past us, and even at an early age, we find ourselves overcommitting to things we "sort of like" and not spending enough time doing the things that truly energize us.

Take a look at your week. Are there things that are not bringing you energy, happiness, and joy that you can consolidate, cancel, or replace? Once you do so, you will have time to add in things that will bring you closer to your goals. This will give you more excitement and energy for each day.

When you begin thinking about your days, please consider a few things. For example, your current career may be both a "need" and a "want" if you love what you do for a living. However, the time you spend volunteering at your child's school might be something you feel obligated to do for others, taking valuable energy away from you. Maybe there is another way you can give back to your child's school, utilizing a different talent you have, without doing something you don't enjoy?

Without taking the time to look at your priorities, you might not have realized how draining some parts of your week are. Could you choose to change things around to add more value and brighten your week?

Look at your schedule every day for the next week or so. Even simple chores that you are responsible for take time: cleaning and maintaining your home, commuting to work, getting enough exercise, taking care of children, volunteering, watching TV, reading books, going to school, etc.

Once you have your list, take a close look at how you actually spend your time. This will give you some insight into how you could spend your time more efficiently. Then, you can make time to do new things that will help you meet your short-term, long-term, and life goals.

Still need to free up more time? Look into taking similar tasks and reorganizing them so that you can do them in blocks, saving you precious time. For example, if you spend time cooking every night, consider instead cooking every other night and making enough for two meals at once.

By eliminating some of the things that take energy away from you, you could create time to fit in workouts, learn new skills, go back to school, or achieve any other goal that you set for yourself.

Know that some things that we need to do can also be things that take energy away from us. *We still need to do them.* If you have a young child, but don't care for changing diapers, remind yourself that it won't last forever. If you (like me) don't love washing dishes, perhaps you can make a deal with your partner or roommate to trade off doing that task.

Sometimes it can be a simple change that makes all the difference.

For some, the simple change of not watching as much television at night can make it easier to wake up earlier, creating time for a morning workout or study time—and bringing them closer to achieving goals that they otherwise would not be able to make time for.

Will it be easy to make all these changes? No, but it can be as simple as prioritizing what is most important to you and gives the most happiness and joy to your days. This can be done in steps. Set these priorities as weekly goals and start making them happen!

Forward Momentum

> *"Arriving at one goal is the starting point to another." ~John Dewey*

Forward momentum is a gift you receive once you complete your first goal. When you do, you will be rewarded with confidence, pride, and excitement—which carries over and gives you the momentum to keep going after your dreams.

Each decision requires us to ask ourselves, "Am I moving closer to, or further away from, my goals?" Momentum gives us a nudge and reminds us that achievement is possible if we continue the fight.

> *"Life is like riding a bicycle. To keep your balance, you must keep moving." ~Albert Einstein*

When you are about to complete a goal, it is the perfect time to define another. By setting your next goal before completing the other, you will constantly have something to work toward and keep you moving forward. We all have goals—to finish a degree, become lighter, get in better shape, change careers, have a child. For most of us, it will take several smaller goals achieved back-to-back in order to get to the final result.

For instance, to finish a long-term goal of completing an unfinished college degree, it is great to have a smaller goal of achieving B or higher grades for each semester. Even weekly goals of completing and turning in your homework on time will move you closer to receiving your degree. Creating time to study and attend classes while working or taking care of a family should be included in your goal details.

Finding ways to keep you motivated and excited for each new set of goals will get you past the finish line. A successful school semester means you are one step closer to goal completion. You aren't going to wait until you finish one class before registering for the next one. Instead, get near the end of the class and then commit to the next step in your journey.

Positive pressure will bring forward momentum. That is exactly what you need to make all your dreams a reality.

The most important thing is to get started. Take the leap, dive into the deep end, and go for it. Make the first step by writing down your goals and the details of what you need to accomplish them.

Then, break your bigger goals down into manageable short-term goals, complete each set on time, and soon enough, you will be celebrating your victory. The key is to not get overwhelmed. If you feel like you need help, ask for it.

SECTION TWO

BELIEVE

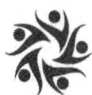

"Many of life's failures

are people who did not realize

how close they were to success

when they gave up."

~Thomas Edison

INSPIRATION OR DESPERATION?

"Believe in yourself and all that you are. Know that there is something inside you that is greater than any obstacle." ~Christian D. Larson

For most people, change occurs when there is either great inspiration or great desperation. Which do you consider to be the motivation for you to change? Or is it a combination of both?

For me, change began when I was feeling despair and desperation, but what launched me full speed ahead into change was a source of inspiration that I never expected.

One day, while I was in physical therapy for my spine injury, I was prescribed the use of an elliptical machine for two minutes— my goal for the entire session. As I was getting on the machine, my doctor walked into the training room with a female athlete and two men whose jackets had Olympic rings on them.

I knew my spine specialist, an endurance athlete himself, worked with several Olympic teams. There were framed photos of Olympian athletes hanging on the walls. But I didn't expect to see any such athletes in this office, and I certainly didn't expect to see them using the equipment alongside me.

When I had first entered the specialist's office several weeks before, barely walking and overweight, I was already feeling depressed, and I soon felt even worse as I compared myself to this woman, clearly an accomplished athlete. I was just a mom who wanted to take care of herself and her girls, not (at that point) someone looking to become incredibly active, let alone athletically competitive.

I was upset and clearly resentful. My first thoughts about seeing the Olympic group enter the physical therapy room were, "Why would they let a healthy athlete in here? Are they trying to make us all feel worse than we already do?" There was a younger man across from me on a bike, rehabbing his knee from surgery. We glanced at each other with questioning looks.

I also thought, "What could be wrong with her? She seems to be running faster than I have ever seen someone run in all my 39 years." The Olympic men and my doctor were examining her shoulder placement, and it seemed that they were concluding that the height of her right shoulder was a tiny bit higher than her left. I bitterly thought, "Could that really be slowing her down? Some of us can hardly walk in here!"

Then something happened. I brought myself back into the present, and for a brief moment of clarity, was able to see the situation for what it was: I was in the presence of an amazing athlete, one who I am sure had overcome many obstacles to get to where she now was. Yes, she was fast, and she didn't appear to be injured, but clearly *she was*. No matter the level of help that she needed, she deserved to be there as much as I did.

In that moment, I took a deep breath and asked myself "Why not me? Why can't I run like that? Anything is possible, right?" I was in pain, barely moving, sad, and overweight. I felt lost, but in that moment I came alive. I was able to take a moment of desperation and turn it into inspiration through gratitude. I finished my appointment that day and left with a smile on my face and a story in my heart.

"It is never too late to be what you might have been." ~George Eliot

What is *your* story? How does it direct you on the path you are beginning? Take some time to be present and see where you are coming from—inspiration or desperation. Either way, know anything is possible.

Am I Ready?

"The moment you doubt whether you can fly, you cease forever to be able to do it." ~Peter Pan (J.M. Barrie)

No one actually sets out to fail. You don't start something with the intention of not finishing—or do you? So many people have good intentions when they begin the journey of accomplishing a new goal or adventure. The problem comes when you don't fully plan for the "what ifs" and the resistance you will encounter, and when you don't know the reason "why" you are doing it.

By the end of this book you will have enough confidence to move forward with any goal of any size. However, you will still have to do the work; I cannot do it for you. After all, that is where the pride of accomplishment comes from: when you accomplish challenging things on your own.

When you achieve your goal, you will feel like you are floating on air. The actual end point will feel good, but knowing what you had to give up or crowd out in order to get there is what you will most honor yourself for.

"Do one thing every day that scares you." ~Eleanor Roosevelt

At what point will the courage to take a leap to achieve your dreams more than outweigh the pain of staying the same? Is that time *now*? If not, what would have to align in order for you to trust yourself and go for it? What will it take to make you want change?

Becoming self-aware enough to make tough decisions is what you need in order to accomplish any goal. If the above questions are challenging for you to answer, then you are on the right track. If they were easy to answer, you would have already achieved your goals. There has been something that has held you back from each of them. Now is the time to discover what that thing is for you and move past it in order to truly live.

Are you ready to take the leap and go after your dreams?

You are ready when the difficulties at work outweigh the fear of making a bold change to a new industry. When the pain of disease or being overweight outweighs the challenge of getting up early to work out. When returning to school and realizing your lifelong goal of finishing your degree outweighs the fear of not being good enough to succeed. When the heartbreak of not going after a big dream outweighs the challenges you might face in order to achieve it. That is when big dreams and goals are accomplished.

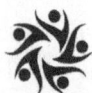

Don't Wait to Make a Change

"Why do you stay in prison when the door is so wide open?" ~Rumi, as interpreted by Coleman Barks

When we think of the word *change,* most of our thoughts are usually fear-based.

Do you have to hit bottom to change? How can you make the leap when you don't know how far you have to go?

The truth is, you can't know how far you need to go, but you do know something: you do NOT want to continue living the way you have been. You also do not want to keep doing what you are currently doing if it doesn't satisfy you.

Life is meant to be about choosing what you love. Life can and should be full of happiness, health, kindness, passion, and the feeling of truly being alive. Everyone's given right is to feel all of these things. There isn't one person who doesn't deserve wonderful things in life. You would not want to keep happiness, love, and joy from a small child, so why do you keep it from yourself? Stop making life so hard for yourself and start believing that you deserve all the great things that are coming your way.

The Rumi quote at the beginning of this section so poignantly reminds us that we are all in control of our own destinies. No matter where you are in your life or what situation you find yourself in, there is always hope. You just need to see it and bring it to yourself. What are you waiting for?

If you don't like your surroundings, why do you choose to stay? If you don't love your career, why do you continue to move forward with it, just barely getting through each day? I see many people fight only when they reach the end of their rope, hit rock bottom, and have nowhere to go but up. But you don't have to wait that long and let life get that bad before you decide to make a change.

What if you chose to engage after your very first moment of clarity? We all have those moments: the times when our heart beats a little faster and we see a small clearing in the clouds. We know that there is always sunshine above every storm-filled sky; we just need to stay focused on that ray of hope until we can further our momentum.

A moment of clarity and hope is the exact time to trust ourselves. Having a goal with clear intentions, knowing your "why," and going after your dreams with a plan can get you where you want to go. No need to be afraid or fear change. Just take a deep breath, and believe. The door is wide open; all you need to do is walk out and create new and exciting opportunities. Create health like you didn't even know was possible, and do things you never imagined in your wildest dreams.

It won't be easy, but it is possible. The best is yet to come!

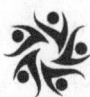

Why, WHY?

"What would you do if you knew you could not fail?" ~Schueller

When you give your goal meaning it comes to life. This is what will keep you going when the going gets tough. This "why" will get you up early in the morning so you can move closer to your goal. It is what will keep you smiling even when people question your motivation. Your "why" is what is most important—not anyone else's thoughts about you and your dreams. After all, the naysayers don't live inside of you; they don't know what you are feeling every day.

Your "why" is personal to you and you alone. It will be your constant underlying motivation so you never stop reaching for your dreams.

When you know without a shadow of a doubt what makes you want to achieve a goal you become unstoppable.

Perhaps your "why" is to feel good in your own skin, to lower your risk of cancer and diabetes, to fulfill a lifelong dream, to show your children what is possible, or any number of other great reasons. When you truly know your "why," the big and small steps you need to take to create a path to achieving it seem so much easier to make.

Take some time to really think about your "why." When it is clear, your chances of achieving your goal become so much greater. Having well-thought-out reasons why we want to achieve our goals sets ourselves up for success.

I have every client print several copies of his "why" and put a copy in his journal, on his mirror, in his car, in his gym bag, and in his wallet. I even have each client take a picture of his "why" to use as the background for his phone or computer. Having your "why" in front of you at all times will keep you laser focused.

Why do you want to accomplish your goal? What benefits will come to you when you accomplish it? What will it feel like to succeed? How will you feel one, two, or five years from now if you choose NOT to go after your goal?

More important than having your goal in front of you is knowing the reasons why you WILL accomplish it. Never lose sight of these very important words.

Positive Pressure

> *"Courage starts with showing up and letting ourselves be seen." ~Brené Brown*

When starting a new adventure toward a goal, sometimes the scariest thing to do is to share our intention with others. We often doubt ourselves due to failed past attempts, and choose not to share our excitement with others in the future. After all, it is one thing to let ourselves down, but another to let down all those we care about.

But when we begin to share with our family, friends, and co-workers—and yes, this includes posting on social media—our goals become real. Not just real to *us*, but also to others. Whether or not others understand why we are choosing to go after a goal, it is ours, and we need to hold fast to our desire to achieve it.

By sharing intentions with those you care about—and taking it a step further to tell them when you will achieve your goals—you give yourself the gift of positive pressure. This is one of my favorite success strategies.

Asking for help from those around you is a wonderful resource. The people you ask don't necessarily have to do anything, but it is human nature that when we tell another we are committing to accomplishing a certain goal, we then feel obligated to do it. Move past the nervousness and uncertainty and take a leap. Believe in YOU and share your goals with all.

I will be the first to tell you that sharing your goals, dreams, and intentions publicly can be challenging. Even after practicing it for years, I still have a moment of hesitation before I press "post" or "send." Then I take a deep breath and remember that everything I have accomplished up until now happened because I was brave enough to share my intentions with others. Positive pressure works.

I give myself a gift: the gift of motivation, the gift of belief in myself, and the gift of possibility.

Who are you going to share your intentions with today? Take some time to send a message, or call someone who cares for you, and tell them how you are going to accomplish your dream!

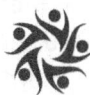

Be Brave

*"Do not go where the path may lead, go
instead where there is no path and leave
a trail." ~Ralph Waldo Emerson*

When we go after the things we love, desire, and are truly passionate about, we need to do so with bold abandonment. It isn't about winning or losing, but believing that achievement is possible. Nothing amazing is ever done without trying. Those who believe that something is not possible not only don't achieve their hopes, but often live to see the day when someone else who *did* believe succeeded in their place. Don't let that be you.

For years, no one believed it was possible to run a mile in under four minutes. Most runners stopped trying to break the record after several failed attempts. But it only took one man, an Englishman named Robert Bannister, to believe in himself enough to break the record. In 1954 he ran a mile in three minutes and 59.4 seconds. That translates to over 15 miles an hour. Hard to even imagine what that would look like! Yet, his record only lasted for 46 days. Once he showed the world that it was possible, others began to believe as well. Since then, the "four-minute barrier" has been broken by many athletes, and the record has been lowered by almost 17 seconds.[4]

Many like to follow, but very few are brave enough to blaze a new trail—one that no one else thought was possible—as Robert Bannister did. He believed before anyone else. And he also trained like no one had trained before in order to accomplish this task. He was focused and did everything in his power to prepare himself mentally and physically to achieve his dream. Others just kept doing the same things and getting the same results. Which type of person are you going to be—one who follows others, or one who dreams of things no one even imagines possible and goes after them?

"It is not the critic who counts; not the man who points out how the strong man stumbles, or where the doer of deeds could have done them better. The credit belongs to the man who is actually in the arena, whose face is marred by dust and sweat and blood; who strives valiantly; who errs, who comes short again and again, because there is no effort without error and shortcoming; but who does actually strive to do the deeds; who knows great enthusiasms, the great devotions; who spends himself in a worthy cause; who at the best knows in the end the triumph of high achievement, and who at the worst, if he fails, at least fails while daring greatly, so that his place shall never be with those cold and timid souls who neither know victory nor defeat." ~Theodore Roosevelt

Daring greatly, whether you achieve "victory or defeat," will give you the confidence to try again and again. The pride that you will earn from truly going after what you trust and believe in will make you a winner no matter what. The important thing to remember is this: if you never try, you will never know what is possible.

Be brave. If you try, you will not only have the opportunity to succeed, but you will receive more knowledge even if you are sidetracked or derailed. This knowledge will help you go after it with a different approach when you begin again tomorrow.

Whether you are supported by those who believe or not, if *you* believe, never stop believing. Remind yourself daily that you deserve this amazing gift you are giving yourself: the gift of life, of truly living and being who you know you deserve to be.

I dare you to be brave, be bold, and BELIEVE!

Trust Your Instincts

"Intuition is seeing with the soul." ~Dean Koontz

Life gives us many signals. First, it is a tap on the shoulder; then it is a pebble, a rock, or, heaven forbid, a brick. Human beings are feeling individuals who must trust their instincts. That gut reaction when we just *know* something is wrong is our true voice. We need to trust it.

Open your eyes and your heart. When you overhear a conversation, see something on the news, or hear a song on the radio that resonates with you, trust that those messages were meant for you. I don't believe in coincidences. You were meant to hear them.

Yet often, we dismiss these signals. We believe there is no way they could be for us. More often than not, we never even hear or see them. We are so busy thinking about what happened in the past, worrying about what people think, or contemplating what will occur in the future that we are not living a fully present life.

We are all guilty of looking down at our electronic devices. Whether we are in the car or at home, we tend to always have music playing in the background. We talk more than we listen. Sometimes we like to be distracted so that we don't have to think about the things in our life that we do not love. We constantly have background noise on, when what our bodies really need is some quiet time each day in order to be able to take in life's messages.

Next time you are waiting in line, walking through the park, exercising, or being still, choose to be quiet with no distractions. Don't check your email or social media feeds while waiting. Instead, disconnect and see what you can hear and learn about yourself.

We have to be willing to be quiet and have an open mind. Being clearly in the present, without anything else on our minds, allows us to receive these signals. Ever been waiting in line at a store, overheard a conversation near you, and instantly remembered something that you needed to get done or been reminded of something that you have always wanted to try? That wasn't by accident. That was life giving you clear signals. These are the times when you wish you had a "rewind" button so you could replay what you just saw or heard in order to retain it.

Always be on the lookout for new ideas and thoughts that come your way. This can be a fun way to go through life.

After all, they say life is a gift. Go open it!

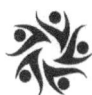

Surrounded by Success

*"Whether you think that you can, or that you
can't, you are usually right." ~Henry Ford*

Surround yourself with people who not only support your
dreams but also push you to continue the fight, and you will
succeed. Our best friends—the ones who know us well—keep us
accountable with positive pressure.

A supportive person isn't someone who enables you to continue
on old paths. No. You can do that all on your own. You want to look
for someone you trust, someone who believes in you.

If you are able to find a coach or friend who has already gone
through what you are about to go through, or is reaching for the
same goal that you are at the same time, that is ideal. She will not
only be there to inspire you with her own success and understand
when the going gets tough, but will also guide you along the way.

Accountability

"If you hang out with chickens, you're going to cluck and if you hang out with eagles, you're going to fly." ~Maraboli

Be willing to ask for help. It does not mean that you are weak, which we unfortunately often tell ourselves. Sometimes society brings on the belief that asking questions or asking for help means weakness. Sometimes it's our own perfectionist tendencies that do this.

Personally, I believe that when I ask for help, that's when I am showing the most strength. To admit to another that I need help or advice gives me the option to learn and decide which help or advice I will choose to take. But when I enter into a situation blindly, because my pride makes me think I already know what I am doing, it can set me in the opposite direction of my goals.

If you don't have a close friend who has been through exactly what you are going through, it might be helpful to instead find a coach to keep you constantly moving forward in the direction of your dreams. An accountability coach will help you see how small steps can lead you to giant leaps forward. I have several coaches, myself: one for my athletic training, and fellow health coaching friends whose advice I call on at times. We all need a sounding board, so find someone to help you get everything out in the open so you can start moving forward. As a coach myself, I love working with people who have anything from small health questions to grand goals.

When you work with a coach, you get to choose what type of accountability works best for you: active or passive. You might choose a weekly call or a daily check-in to discuss your progress; both are good methods to put you on a path to succeed. A coach can also help you decide if your chosen actions are moving you closer to or further away from your goals. No matter what you do during a given day, all things should point in the same direction. Accountability to a coach can make that happen.

A coach or friend can work with you to successfully navigate challenges, resistance, accountability, and planning. He or she can help you discover what will allow you to truly Live Alive Fit (my personal motto and the tagline of my coaching business)— in other words, what will allow you to **live your best life... Alive, Healthy, and Fit**!

Borrow Belief

> *"What's worked for me is not quitting and being passionate about what I do and not giving up— and when I don't believe in myself, turning to others who believe in me." ~Marc Jacobs*

There are going to be times when we lose sight of what we believe in and think we can't go on. At those times, we need to call on others who believe in us and can remind us of what we are capable of. Think of someone who has seen you at your worst but, at the same time, can help remind you what you have already accomplished—someone who wants to follow your journey so he can soon see you at your best.

Be willing to listen and be reminded that you have and will do amazing things.

Find others who share similar goals to you. This might be an online community of like-minded individuals, a school study group, a group exercise class, a coach, a neighbor, or a spouse who wants to join you on your adventure. Get together and share your struggles and wins.

I find that having an accountability group or partner allows me to accomplish more of my goals in a timely fashion. Relying on each other for deadlines and sending each other motivating messages, even short ones, can help keep us moving forward each and every day.

I also find that once friends know about my goals, they can begin to give me accountability. Without even knowing it, they provide me with positive pressure to complete my goals—not just successfully, but on time. When I shared with my extended family that I wanted to complete a 140.6 mile IRONMAN® triathlon, their first response was "Why?" They weren't trying to be combative, although sometimes it seemed that way. I remembered to take a deep breath and share my excitement with them. This showed them all the joys that accomplishing my goal would bring me.

When you are ready to share the news about your exciting goals, make sure that you know exactly why you want to accomplish them, and be ready to ask for—and accept—their support and help.

Healthy Environment

"Surround yourself with people who make you happy. People who make you laugh, who help you when you're in need. People who genuinely care. They are the ones worth keeping in your life. Everyone else is just passing through." ~Karl Marx

Having a healthy living environment is not just about where you live and where you spend your time, but also WHO you surround yourself with.

When we align ourselves with and spend more time around those who have an energy and light we resonate with, it gives us less time to spend with those who bring us down. Each of us are individuals, so the same things will not bring different people joy and true happiness; however, the way certain people live can be replicated.

"Surround yourself with only people who are going to lift you higher." ~Oprah Winfrey

Do your friends find possibility in life, or are they always looking for the worst? Do your family members support health and movement by the way they vacation, live, and spend free time—or do they choose to sit around, eat constantly, and never go outside? Do you yourself choose to be active in your own free time, or do you choose to play video games, watch movies, spend time on the Internet, and sit on the couch?

Take some time to think about where and who you spend your time with during the week. Does your workplace support the choices you make to live your best life? Who do you currently spend time with that makes you feel great? Could you spend more time with them?

This is the environment that will support you and help you move closer to being the best person you can be. You want to make sure it is clean and full of possibility!

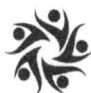

Commitment to You

"Most of the important things in the world have been accomplished by people who have kept on trying when there seemed to be no hope at all." ~Dale Carnegie

Take a close look at your schedule. In the "Small Steps Turn into Giant Leaps" chapter, there is a section called "Making Time for Me." In this section, I encouraged you to find more times during your day to work toward achieving your goal.

Schedule time for yourself. Block out your daily and weekly steps into time slots in your days, and keep those appointments with yourself. Do not give up your time for any reason other than a true emergency. Baking cookies for your child's bake sale, waking up late, or suddenly realizing that it's time to do your taxes are not emergencies; they don't count as reasons to cancel the appointments you've made with yourself.

I know you're busy, but be creative. Could you squeeze in some time for yourself in the early morning so you can check some items off your to-do list? If you schedule time for yourself in the morning, you are more likely to stick to it. In the afternoon, there are more last-minute distractions that could come up.

Remember: keep your commitments to yourself at all costs.

When you are asked if you are free on Wednesday at noon (your pre-scheduled time for *you*) and you say, "I am sorry, I am already booked at that time," you will be surprised what will happen. Nothing! That person will find another time to meet with you. It can be that simple; unfortunately, society has told us that we need to be people pleasers who always say "yes." Always saying yes didn't work for me, and I am sure it isn't working for you either. Like I was, you are probably just saying "no" to yourself every time you say "yes" to someone else.

The bottom line: you never have to give a reason why you won't give up your time. You just don't. If you are compelled to share, you can say something like: "I am an athlete and in training at that time," whether your goal is your first 5k race or a marathon. Or, "I have a class," if you plan to be studying for school.

Remember, be consistent with your commitment to your goal. This is the time you chose for yourself. Don't give in. You and your dreams are very important.

"What's worth doing even if you fail?" ~Brene Brown

When you prioritize what is most important to you and choose which goal you truly want to achieve, it becomes much easier to prioritize your time. Then you can watch your dreams come to life much faster than you could ever have imagined before.

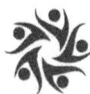

Not If, but When

"Obstacles are those frightful things you see when you take your eyes off your goal." ~Henry Ford

You are moving right along and feeling good about your progress. Week after week, you celebrate small wins and feel the momentum.

All of a sudden, you get sick and are laid out for a week. A family member questions your motive. You have to decide between going on a last-minute business trip or working on your goal. Or, simply, fear of failure overcomes you. What do you do?

The answer is to hang on tight no matter what comes your way. Breathe, believe, and *choose to be* the person you are headed to becoming. Think about how people who have already successfully achieved your goal would react to resistance, setbacks, or fear. They would march right through these obstacles and come out the other side, ready to pick up where they left off.

Do what you can and let go of expectations about the rest. Stay in the present; don't worry about the future; never regret anything from the past. Remember to keep **breathing and believing**.

Your
Comfort
Zone

Where the
magic happens

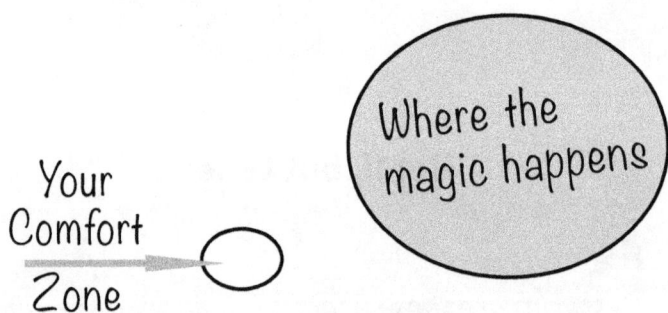

The sooner you get out of your comfort zone, the sooner you will become the person you were meant to be!

Setbacks

"Life is 10 percent what happens to me and 90 percent how I react to it." ~Charles R. Swindoll

Many people believe that when starting down a new path, taking two steps forward and one step back is okay. On my own journey, I usually expect to have constant forward movement, with some detours along the way.

Of course, there will always be things that set us back from time to time. It is how we react to them that matters. If you are driving along and get a flat tire, you don't get a new car. You stop, fix the tire, get back in your car, and keep going.

We get to choose how we react to the good and challenging times that come our way. That is what makes life so great. We get to choose.

It doesn't always seem that simple, but it truly is. I am not asking you to stay positive all the time. We all know that doesn't work. Instead, I want to remind you to think of *what is possible*!

Living a life of gratitude, one that celebrates life's possibilities versus challenges, sets you up for being in a healthy state of mind when unexpected things come your way. You have to believe that you can and will succeed in your endeavors. Stay in a state of gratitude during challenging times. It is possible; you just have to believe.

Resistance

*"Don't be afraid of your fears. They're not there
to scare you. They're there to let you know
that something is worth it." ~C. JoyBell C.*

The greater the resistance, the more important the goal. If it wasn't important to you, there wouldn't be so much opposition; failing would be an option because the outcome wouldn't matter either way. You would just be okay with letting the dream go. But when you truly want something with your whole heart, obstacles come at you fast and furious.

Resistance is like an unwanted friend or a bad four-letter word: it can come in many sizes and forms, and we willingly allow it to overcome us. Author Steven Pressfield, in his book *The War Of Art*, defines resistance as "The Enemy."

*"We can navigate by Resistance, letting it guide us
to that calling or action that we must follow before
all others. Rule of thumb: The more important a
call or action is to our soul's evolution, the more
Resistance we will feel toward pursuing it."[5]*

When you encounter resistance, it is how you choose to confront it that matters. Will you give up? Or will you have your "Why" written down in your pocket, ready to take out so you can remind yourself exactly why you are going after your goal? Those who are prepared for not only *if* but *when* something will occur WILL be ready. When we plan for resistance, from inside us or out, we set ourselves up for success. I once had a friend I would often meet very early in the morning for a workout. I had a habit of texting her to check and see if she was going to make it. I always secretly hoped she would tell me "Go back to bed, we don't need to meet today." Knowing I had this self-sabotaging tendency, I asked for her help. We promised to hold each other accountable and instead send a "get there or else" message before each early morning workout.

Having one-on-one accountability, and our commitment to one another for an entire year, was what helped me learn how to swim. It also helped me to achieve my daily goal of training when I committed to my much larger goal of completing a long-distance triathlon a year later at age forty.

Nonetheless, resistance in many forms came to me every morning. My body screamed at me to go back to bed when the alarm went off, because I was tired. My mind would say "You don't even like to swim. Why go?" I often woke up late and found myself wondering if my friend would notice if I didn't show up.

I set myself up for success by knowing that I needed to push past the resistance and ask for help ahead of time. Being in the pool three times a week by 5:45 a.m., no matter what, was no easy task, but having an accountability partner helped immensely.

If you do not know anyone who is going after a similar goal, introduce yourself to people you run into on your journey toward your goal, and make an effort to get to know others. They could be just like you. Ask how you can support one another. Then, when resistance comes, you will be prepared!

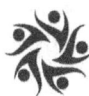

Plan Ahead for "When"

(On being asked how he felt about repeatedly failing to design a working light bulb) "I have not failed. I've just found 10,000 ways that it won't work." ~Thomas Edison

When we check in with ourselves daily, preparing for each day in advance, we set ourselves up for success. Of course, we never know what obstacles might come our way—family or work emergencies, illness, injury. But what we do *most of the time* is what matters.

Prepare for what may come, but don't dwell on it.

It would be a mistake to always be looking over your shoulder for what might come along and hold you back. Instead, focus confidently on controlling the things you *can* control.

When I knew I needed to get up at 5 a.m. for a workout, this self-proclaimed "non-morning person" had to plan ahead the night before by setting out clothes and preparing a protein shake and water bottle—and putting them by the door with my keys, workout bag, shoes, and coat. If I didn't go, I would have to face those items all day long. That created positive pressure to help me get up and go every morning.

Of course, I liked to trick my mind. When the alarm went off, I would bargain with myself: "Just get up and see how you feel." After getting up and seeing my things all ready for me by the door, I'd always say, "Everything is ready, I might as well go." On my way home, I would celebrate my victory, not just because I was getting more fit and moving closer to my goal, but because I had won the mind game with myself. I *was* a morning person, as long as I told myself so.

Having too large of goals can make some of us more likely to quit, so make sure you take your long-term goals and break them down into manageable weekly and daily tasks. This creates momentum that you can use to achieve your complete goals.

Ask yourself, what do I need to do tomorrow, and each day this week, to move me closer to my goal? What do I need to do by the end of the week to move me closer to my goal? What can I do ahead of time to ensure that I accomplish my goals in a timely manner and hold my commitment to myself? By answering these questions, you will set yourself up for success.

Every Sunday night, take some time to create a list of tasks for the week ahead. You can use the action steps in the back of this book as a guide. By doing so, not only will you be more organized, but you will also be able to avoid last-minute changes that could cut into the time that you had set aside for your goal.

Think of some things you could do to set yourself up for success. For instance, if you have a fitness or health goal, cooking large quantities of healthy items one day a week and dividing them into smaller meals could help get you through a busy week and save you lots of time. All of these little things will add up to move you closer to accomplishing your goals instead of letting life take your time away.

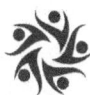

Fear

"Courage is not the absence of fear, but rather the judgment that something else is more important than fear." ~Ambrose Redmoon

Fear is something that everyone feels. But knowing where fear comes from can remove the power that it holds over us. When we acknowledge fear, it takes over our life. When we surrender to its forces, we are immediately stopped in our tracks. No longer can we move forward or even breathe. We are held captive by our own minds.

So what can we do to move past fear? The truth is, we can't. Instead, we have to move right through it. Not past, over, or around it—that only gives it more power. Look fear in the eye and walk straight toward it.

This week, in what ways will you choose to stare your fear in the eye, accomplishing steps toward your goal despite uncomfortable feelings? How good will it feel when you overcome the feelings of resistance and do what you need to in order to live your best life by going after your goals?

"You can conquer almost any fear if you will only make up your mind to do so. For remember, fear doesn't exist anywhere except in the mind." ~Dale Carnegie

Remove the power that fear holds over you. Visualize your fear as a tiny dot, a small insignificant thing that wants to hold you back from your most precious dreams. If fear was calling your child names or being mean to your mother, you would have no problem walking over to it and telling it how you feel, right? So why is your reaction any different when fear is bullying *you*?

You cannot let anyone or anything hold you back from discovering who you were meant to be. Fight and push forward by any means possible.

Take some time now to think about what might be holding you back from accomplishing your goals. What ideas in your head are stopping you in your tracks and making it seem impossible for you to move forward? When you think about achieving your goals, what feelings immediately come to mind? From whom do you feel the most resistance when you attempt certain tasks toward accomplishing your goal?

Nothing worthwhile is ever going to be easy to achieve, and that includes conquering your fears.

Believe in yourself. Believe in yourself. BELIEVE.

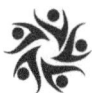

SECTION THREE

BECOME

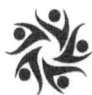

"Consult not your fears

but your hopes and your dreams.

Think not about your frustrations,

but about your unfulfilled potential.

Concern yourself not with what you tried and failed in,

but with what it is still possible for you to do."

~Pope John XXIII

See It, Believe It

*"Your chances of success in any undertaking can
always be measured by your belief in yourself."*
~Robert Collier

What we say, do, and see in our minds will manifest into reality. When we truly believe in what we set out to achieve, and want it with our whole heart, in time it will appear. Sometimes things will appear in our lives a bit differently than we originally planned or envisioned, but they will come if we are patient and diligent with our belief.

There are many techniques that I have used to bring beautiful and amazing things into my life. I am grateful to be able to share them with you. Some of the challenges I have overcome:

- Becoming eighty pounds lighter

- Going from hardly walking to running and being an elite racer

- Learning to swim in my late thirties in order to finish a 140.6 mile ultra-distance triathlon

- Transforming my finances from overspending to budgeted

- Healing spine injuries without surgery

All of these accomplishments came with a tremendous amount of work. I had to learn to be patient. I often needed to become single-focused and learn what I needed to let go of to achieve these goals.

Remember, achieving our goals doesn't always happen on the timeline or in the way we expect. Some of my own challenges took me beyond my expectations, but I always remained open to change and willing to create a better life for myself. By doing so, I overcame what I needed to in order to achieve my goals.

Now it is your turn to use these techniques to become the person you BELIEVE is possible.

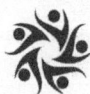

Thoughts Become Reality

"Every thought is a seed. If you plant crab apples, don't count on harvesting Golden Delicious." ~Bill Meyer

Every single thought that we have, either good or bad, will manifest in our lives. Choose to spend your time, thoughts, and energy on what you want, not on what you don't want.

If you are headed to a job you aren't crazy about, approach it with the attitude that today will be the best day ever. If you want to become a fast runner, don't tell yourself it is okay just to jog for now. Instead, create a mantra to repeat as you run: tell yourself that you are fast, light, and strong, no matter what speed you are currently running at.

If you want to be a manager at your organization, don't tell yourself that you would be okay with someone else getting the job. Instead, walk in the door with confidence, like you own the place, and take pride in everything you do. Lead by example, and soon enough others will see you as a leader.

If you want to get straight A's in school, don't tell yourself that a B every once in a while is okay. Instead, make time to study, create an action plan, and walk into each test with confidence, knowing that you studied hard and will do great.

"The happiness of your life depends upon the quality of your thoughts: therefore, guard accordingly, and take care that you entertain no notions unsuitable to virtue and reasonable nature." ~Marcus Aurelius

Start telling yourself what you want to hear. Say it out loud so that you don't just hear it in your head, but hear yourself actually say it. Repetition sets it in your mind as a new song you can play.

Use words with possibility in all of your everyday conversations. Instead of "I could, I have to, I might," use "I will, I get to, and I can" in order to give hope to your goals. Even when I was struggling to learn to swim at the age of 38—and I didn't like having to swim in the very early mornings—I would wake up every day and say "I AM a swimmer," and "I GET to go swim this morning." Just six months later I was able to swim a mile nonstop in open water, without the security of a pool. I believed I would and became what I chose.

Some say "Fake it 'til you make it." I say, BELIEVE IT and you will BECOME IT!

It was challenging to keep forging forward when I really did not want to continue. But I knew my goal and what I needed to do to get to it, and I moved forward daily in the direction of my dreams to achieve it. Achieving your goals and realizing your dreams is truly a choice.

Take charge of your life. Use your words to command your brain's attention. Tell yourself what you will achieve in life.

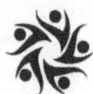

I AM...

*"I am the greatest, I said that even before
I knew I was." ~Muhammad Ali*

When you believe with all your heart that you are already who you want to become, your mind can't tell the difference. I use a few empowering words to keep me focused during tough times in my life. When I am challenged while training or racing, I constantly repeat my mantra over and over again until I am refocused on what I need to do: "I AM light, I AM fast, I AM strong, I BELIEVE."

Take some time right now and write down a few words that make you feel amazing. Each day, schedule time to say this mantra. Any time you feel out of sorts, you can bring yourself right back to a good place in your head by calling on these words. Close your eyes and say them out loud. Repeat your words, several times in a row, at a rhythmic pace.

Take a moment, clear your mind, and take a few deep cleansing breaths. Then, remember a time when you accomplished something amazing that wasn't easy.

Now open your eyes and write down whatever came into your mind. Don't edit yourself. Just let the words flow in any order and on any place on your page. This is who you ARE and who you will fully become when you choose to believe it. Have fun dreaming!

Visualize to Become

"Visualize this thing that you want, see it, feel it, believe in it. Make your mental blueprint, and begin to build." ~Robert Collier

With each thought, each breath, the way we carry ourselves, and the way we live, we must believe we are already who we want to become.

When I first thought about walking a half-marathon, I doubted myself before I even began. I was inspired by my then seven-year-old daughter, who asked me if I would walk with her while she trained for a children's marathon at her school. If she could be an "athlete," so could I.

As soon as I started to call myself an "athlete," I began to eat how I thought athletes should eat. I carried myself like I thought an athlete would, stood taller, and took care of myself better.

I created a training plan and walked several times a week. I walked everywhere. I walked to the post office, to the store, to do errands. I believed I could finish that 13.1 miles before I even began it.

When I got to the starting line of the race, I had already visualized what it would be like to cross the line at the finish. I could see that image and used it along with the love I could feel from those who supported me. That kept me moving for hours. I had hardly been able to walk out my door just seven months before, but now I was walking a three-hour half-marathon.

"Everything you can imagine is real." ~Pablo Picasso

Ever since that day, I have used visualization to get everything that I currently have in my life. Even while I was writing this book, I could see the finished manuscript sitting right in front of me.

When I first raced a duathlon (run, bike, run) at the USA Age Group National Championships (only my second time doing a duathlon), I saw myself finishing strong. I knew it was going to be tough, since I wasn't the strongest runner there, but I went for it and gave it everything I had, and I placed twentieth. While only the top 18 runners automatically qualified for the Age Group World Championships, I held onto the belief that I would get there. I received a message just one week later asking me to join Team USA and represent the United States, as a top age group athlete, in Spain.

"I dream my painting and I paint my dream." ~Vincent van Gogh

Seven months later, my two daughters and husband got to watch me race with the best in the world on an international scale. Everyone was screaming "Go USA" as I ran by—a dream I thought would never come true, even though as a young child, I had dreamed of being on the gymnastics or ice skating USA Team, as many young girls do.

You never know when your dreams will manifest in a different form, so hold on to them, and keep them close to your heart. Even a 42-year-old mother of two can represent her country with pride and gratitude in her heart.

Nothing can stop us from achieving those things that we BELIEVE are possible for ourselves.

"I Deserve" to Be Happy

"Any thought that is passed on to the subconscious often enough and convincingly enough is finally accepted." ~Robert Collier

Not only do you deserve happiness, you are worth all the time and energy that you spend taking care of yourself. I used to feel so selfish for taking time away from my family to exercise, paint, or take a class that truly inspired me. But now I know that spending some of my time this way is the best choice I can make for myself and my family. When I come home full of energy, I am fully present, focused, and ready to spend quality time with the ones I love.

"Finish each day and be done with it. You have done what you could. Some blunders and absurdities no doubt crept in; forget them as soon as you can. Tomorrow is a new day. You shall begin it serenely and with too high a spirit to be encumbered with your old nonsense." ~Ralph Waldo Emerson

One of my favorite reminders is one that anyone who has flown on an airplane has heard, but it is worth repeating here: "Put on your own oxygen mask first, then assist those around you." We often want to give up on ourselves and use any last bit of energy on helping others. But self-care brings us more joy, passion, and energy for life. If we do not take care of ourselves first—including our spirit and our soul—we will not have enough energy to give anything back to those we love and care for.

When we choose to go on a walk, give ourselves quiet time alone, take a fitness class, or participate in anything else that fuels us or puts us into a more balanced state, we are doing it selflessly. We will be able to love deeper, feel stronger, give more energy, and be more alive and present for those we love.

What do you deserve to be in your life? Happy? Joyful? In love? Passionate? Successful in a career you enjoy? Healthy?

Make a declaration to yourself and repeat it daily if needed: "I deserve..." And don't stop until you know deep in your heart that what you desire is also what you deserve.

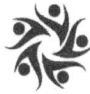

L O V E

noun \'lǝv
1a (1) : strong affection for another arising out of
kinship or personal ties <maternal love for a child>
(2) : attraction based on sexual desire : affection
and tenderness felt by lovers (3) : affection based on
admiration, benevolence, or common interests <love
for his old schoolmates>

1b : an assurance of affection <give her my love>

2: warm attachment, enthusiasm, or devotion <love
of the sea.

3a: the object of attachment, devotion, or admiration
<baseball was his first love> 3b (1): a beloved person:
darling—often used as a term of endearment (2)
British— used as an infomral term of address[6]

Love is not only a feeling or a way to define a relationship, but also a way to show enthusiasm or devotion for things and situations. Love has a way of binding similar people with common interests together.

The more I spend time feeling and sharing love, the more I want to teach others how it can help them. I lived for years with a lack of love. Don't get me wrong; I had a wonderful husband who loved me no matter my body size or career choice. I had two beautiful girls who gave me unconditional love each day. I have four sisters and a brother, along with parents who have been married for over fifty years and share their love freely. From the outside, I clearly have never had a lack of love. However, at one time I wasn't able to accept it. I didn't like who I was or where my life was headed. You might feel that way now.

You have the opportunity to create more love in your life and the ability to receive more love not only from the people in your life, but your surrounding environment. I now find love in many small things in life: the opportunity to purchase organic fruits and vegetables, clean drinking water, and sunlight streaming through my home windows. But, I also find love in larger things, like my family and a career that brings me more joy than I knew was possible.

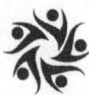

Why Love?

"Wheresoever you go, go with all your heart." ~Kongzi

Love has a far greater power than many of us choose to give it. When we say we love something, and truly feel this love from within ourselves, a chemical reaction occurs in our brain. We place value on that item, person, or activity. That value is then recorded in our minds and hearts for future reference. Each time we hear, think, or see anything about the thing or person we love, that same positive, amazing reaction occurs in our mind and heart.

"How do you spell 'love'?" ~Piglet

"You don't spell it... you feel it." ~Pooh, A.A. Milne

Life can throw us many curveballs, but if we know what we love, we can call upon those things or people in our times of need.

Years ago I had a job that particularly challenged me. I had a long commute and was surrounded by negative co-workers every day. So I began to use an exercise to recite what I loved. On my drive to work, instead of complaining to myself about the traffic and how I couldn't wait to be headed home again—even though I hadn't even arrived at work yet—I would recite all of the things I loved.

I would turn the radio off and repeat, out loud, over and over again, the things that I loved in that moment: "I love the trees. I love the way the light reflects on the lake. I love fresh air. I love the sun shining on my face. I love the song playing right now. I love this car that transports me safely." When the immediate ones were seemingly done, I would remember to love all sorts of other things in my life: "I love my daughters. I love my husband. I love traveling. I love hugs. I love the color red. I love my home. I love to paint. I love life. I love to run. I love my friends," and so on.

I spent my entire drive to work reciting what I loved. This put me in a better mood and made my day go by so much faster. I chose to do it every single day until I could secure a new job closer to home that I enjoyed. I still use this technique to get me through challenging situations that come my way and times when I need a pick-me-up. It works. I dare you to try it.

When I felt stuck in my life, love made each day bearable. Love made me focus on the good in my life instead of on things I didn't care for. Love made me a better person, a better employee, a better friend, wife, mother, and sister. I liked who I was when I chose to use love as a tool to get through very challenging times.

Always remember to acknowledge what you love every morning, at lunch, on walks, and in your car. Always compliment things you like about those around you. The things you love don't have to mean much to others, but they do need to mean something to you. This is how you bring more of what you love right back to yourself.

"It is good to love many things, for therein lies the true strength, and whosoever loves much performs much, and can accomplish much, and what is done in love is well done." ~Vincent van Gogh

Take a few moments and say out loud all of the things you love. Some are probably obvious ("my dear friends who support my goals"); some are simple ("fresh food to eat"); some are subtle ("clean water to drink"). But they are all important if they give you joy.

Use this exercise any time you need to be uplifted. It can be done verbally or in writing. Give it a try—you will be grinning from ear to ear before this exercise is over. If you're not, keep going. Love brings love.

Gratitude

"Gratitude opens the door to... the power, the wisdom, the creativity of the universe. You open the door through gratitude." ~Deepak Chopra

Sometimes I don't feel like I have much to be grateful for. Some days, it is all I can do to be grateful for fresh air, clean water, and a roof over my head. But those things are more than many in the world have.

Even in times of great challenge with my weight and physical pain, I was grateful to have a husband who could help me out of bed. I was grateful for children who I loved and for a car that could take me where I needed to go.

Every day brings new feelings of gratitude. Some are grand and glorious examples of how much we love and are loved, and how we have things to love in our lives. Other days, we just feel like getting by. Either way, clear and constant gratitude for all you are, have, and do will help you continue to move forward in life.

Being grateful forces us to see what is possible and what could be. We are reminded of what is good in the world and what we hope to have more of.

"Gratitude is not only the greatest of virtues, but the parent of all others." ~Cicero (106-43 BC), *Roman philosopher, statesman, and orator*

It is critical that we have gratitude for all things and people in our lives. The power of the words "thank you" are underestimated by most. However, when we are given those words as a special gift, we are reminded of what they truly mean, and hopefully that will inspire others to share them more.

Giving for Life

*"Blessed are those that can give without remembering
and receive without forgetting." ~Elizabeth Bibesco*

Life is what we make of it. You have the opportunity to bring more love into your life than you ever knew was possible. Ever have someone you didn't even know compliment you on something you were wearing or doing? What kind of instantaneous joy did that bring to your day? The unconditional love of kindness, compassion, and affection is a type of love that I really resonate with, which is why I find small ways each day to bring a little love into the lives of strangers.

*"The true measure of a man is how he treats someone
who can do him absolutely no good." ~Samuel Johnson*

Two Purdue University students called "The Compliment Guys" gained national attention when they set out to give free compliments to other students every Wednesday afternoon on campus. With no intention of gaining anything in return, Brett Westcott and Cameron Brown launched a very polite practice of complimenting complete strangers as they passed by, and it has turned into something viral. Now, other college campuses are encouraging similar behavior.

"I love giving free compliments—there's nothing else I'd rather do," Westcott told the *Purdue University News*. The more they give back to their community, the more it encourages others to do the same. That is an amazing gift, and it doesn't cost a penny. Brown says, "The whole goal is to brighten people's days."

Imagine your life if you chose to include the simple act of complimenting a few people each day. It doesn't have to be anything outrageous, and you don't have to spend money to give a few kind words—even a genuine smile can work.

Giving is so much better than receiving when it is done without any thought of gain or return.

When you choose to give, you might find that you will be rewarded in ways you can't imagine: you will start receiving love and happiness from more unexpected places than you thought possible. Go ahead, give it a try.

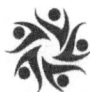

Attraction

"What we are today comes from our thoughts of yesterday. And our present thoughts build our life of tomorrow. Our life is the creation of our mind." ~Buddha

Attraction can work in a few ways. One way is by knowing that what you give out, you will receive back in some form or another. The other way attraction can work is that you will be drawn to those with similar thoughts and ideas as yourself. This is called "the law of attraction," a belief that stems from the notion that "like attracts like." Knowing that both people and their thoughts are made of "pure energy," it makes sense that by focusing on positive or negative thoughts, you can bring more of the same energy as a result.

The most important thing to remember about the law of attraction is this: What you give out in your thoughts, actions, and energy, you will attract more of. This concept works for both positive and negative thoughts when it comes to attracting people, scenarios, and things into your life.

Have you ever had a challenging day where it seemed easier to complain to everyone instead of letting it go, only to have even more challenging things come your way? You were giving bad energy to those challenges, so you attracted even more chaos to your life. Remember, you are always going to receive back the same type of energy you give out.

When we choose to complain about or dwell on things that are not healthy for us and don't give us good energy (for instance, thoughts of possibility, joy, or love), we bring more of them our way. If you instead encourage yourself to think of what is possible and envision hope for the future and a desire to create your best life, you will attract scenarios and others who feel and desire the same as you. That is the law of attraction working in you. Anything truly is possible.

"Whatever relationships you have attracted in your life at this moment, are precisely the ones you need in your life at this moment. There is a hidden meaning behind all events, and this hidden meaning is serving your own evolution." ~Deepak Chopra

When we spend quality time with individuals who are fully present, happy, joyful, and honestly loving life, we often feel all those wonderful attributes as well. When we allow ourselves to be open to the possibility of change, it tends to lift us up.

But when we spend time with people who bring us down, do not have our best intentions in mind, or are sad or depressed, we begin to take on their feelings. The only way to combat this negativity is to have our own energy be so high, and full of love and life, while in their presence that we are able to separate ourselves from them emotionally. Most people do not last long in a negative environment without experiencing a drain of their own energy. When you choose the type of environment you want to spend time in, keep this in mind.

You can test this theory next time you go to an event with a bunch of people you do not know well. Walk in like you have had your best day ever, and believe it with your entire being. Truly be grateful, kind, and gracious to everyone. Then notice who you are attracted to and who strikes up conversations with you. Is it the people on the couch who seem to be unhappy with their current lives, or do you find yourself moving toward those who are smiling, seem to enjoy life, and are carefree and fully present?

We attract those who are similar to ourselves, so start spending more time with people who have attributes you hope to achieve through change in your own life. Have fun with it.

What Is Possible

"Start by doing what's necessary; then do what's possible; and suddenly you are doing the impossible."
~Francis of Assisi

We place ceilings on our dreams far lower than we ever should. If we could only open up the facade and see that the true ceiling is so much higher, our confidence would grow ten-fold. The sky is the limit when it comes to what you choose to accomplish. Truly it is.

So why don't more of us realize this? We are conditioned from a very early age that failure is not an option, so we learned to only commit to doing things that we were pretty sure we could achieve.

We do not often think about what might occur if we dream bigger.

When we go big, we might need to course-correct or make adjustments at some point. But what will happen if you *do* achieve that dream goal? Your life will never be the same. You will be doing things that others never dreamed were even possible, living the life you desire, and likely sharing that energy, inspiration, and joy with others.

Don't you think that the possibility of a positive outcome far outweighs the risk that you might have to try more than once to achieve it? I do, but that might be because I have taken big risks with several of the goals that I have achieved, and had them pay off. I wouldn't take even one moment of that time spent in challenge, fear, or resistance back.

"What you get by achieving your goals is not as important as what you become by achieving your goals." ~Zig Ziglar

You will need to put in the work and spend time each day visualizing yourself already where you want to be, but it will all be worth it in the end. Do not let other people's thoughts about what is possible affect what you choose to go after. Others don't get to choose your life path for you; you do. Calmly tell them that you appreciate their advice, but only you know what is best for you.

And trust that when you accomplish your amazing goal, you will be inspiring those people who did not think you could (or would) do it, and showing everyone that you not only believe in yourself, but that you truly can do anything you put your heart into.

Does this mean I want you to quit your job and go after your big dream without any thought or plan? No, but in time, while you continue to believe what is possible, and complete steps that will bring you closer to your dream, you can make the leap with more confidence. It won't be easy, but it can be simple. Be patient, and it will come.

Happiness Brings Health

"Happiness is the meaning and the purpose of life, the whole aim and end of human existence." ~Aristotle

By knowing exactly why you want it, working through specific steps to get it, and knowing what it will bring you when you achieve it, your happiness is imminent.

The wonderful part is that by achieving even your smaller weekly goals, you will begin to shine. Each success piles on top of the last. With accountability, you will be encouraged to continue the climb. It is only a matter of time before you reach your goal.

"The purpose of life is the expansion of happiness." ~Maharishi Mahesh Yogi

Once you have achieved your dream goal, you will not only have more joy and happiness, but you will physically change as well. Your body is constantly changing, whether you realize it or not. You might have heard that your body regenerates organs and cells, but you might not have thought about how this scientific principle could affect you. In fact, you have the opportunity to completely change the entire makeup of your body in just one year.

Dr. Masaru Emoto, a researcher and alternative healer from Japan, amassed a good deal of evidence about the magic of positive thinking. He became famous for his water molecule experiments in 2004, demonstrating "that human thoughts and intentions can alter physical reality, such as the molecular structure of water." [7] In fact, the human body is comprised of at least 60 percent water, so Emoto's research has poignant implications about the power of positive thinking.

Another of Emoto's experiments used rice to demonstrate how destructive negative thinking can be, and how positive thinking holds power. He placed a portion of cooked rice in two separate containers, labeling one "thank you" and the other "you fool." He then positioned the containers of rice publicly in a school and asked the children to read the labels out loud every time they passed by. Thirty days later, the rice that was told the positive thought ("thank you") had barely changed, while the rice that was told the negative thought ("you fool") was moldy and rotten.

What can we take from Emoto's studies? By living with greater joy, love, gratitude, and happiness, you are choosing to give yourself greater health, because your actions and words actually change the physical makeup of your body. We get to choose how we treat ourselves and others. Now that you know some of the implications, you might choose your words more wisely.

Can you imagine wanting to get up each day because you can't wait to get to work? Or receiving a steady, generous paycheck for doing something you love? It just takes one leap of faith to begin the process, and a commitment to seeing the worth in every moment of the challenging work you will be putting in.

You are so close to becoming the person you have always dreamed of.

Happiness and health, along with joy and excitement for each new day, are just a few of the things that will come to you as you begin to achieve your goals. With each success, you will increase your momentum and your desire to continue on the path to become the person you were meant to be.

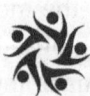

Anything

"People say nothing is impossible,
but I do nothing every day."
~Pooh, A.A. Milne

Anything you picture yourself accomplishing, you can achieve. When you visualize your goal, your mind can see that it is already possible. If you couldn't imagine it, then it would be far more challenging to achieve.

What we say, do, and see in our minds will manifest into reality. When we truly believe in what we set out to do or achieve, then it cannot help but become so. Sometimes things will appear in our lives a bit differently than we originally planned or envisioned, but they *will* appear.

After I became active, I dreamed of running in the Boston marathon, a challenging race to qualify for. I was on track with my training. I ran each day and worked very hard at attaining more speed. But just a few months away from my qualifying race, I developed knee pain which forced me to drop out of the race. To rehabilitate my knee, I was led to cycling. What I hadn't realized was that I had been running mainly because I wanted to be challenged and fulfilled, and cycling began to fill that need for me.

The cycling I did for therapy led me to my next career as a cycling coach and top age-group racer. I had never ridden longer than a few miles in my life; now I ride almost daily and accomplish routes on my bike that I don't even like to drive in a car. Life often brings us gifts that appear differently than we envision at first—but are still good things.

"When you do what you fear most, then you can do anything." ~Stephen Richards

Take on something greater than you believe you might be able to accomplish. This doesn't necessarily mean that you should set an unrealistic goal of running a marathon in sixty days if you aren't even running a mile now. However, I do think that giving yourself an inspiring goal—like running a marathon in one year, with a half-marathon goal eight to nine months from now, and a five-kilometer event in two to three months—is absolutely possible.

On the other hand, if you choose a goal too easy to achieve, it might not be worth achieving, which makes it easy to get distracted off the path. So, go after a dream and goal that inspires you—one that makes you excited and nervous at the same time just thinking about it.

Even if you have to give up some time and activities during your week to achieve your goal, you will be so proud of yourself when you achieve it. You can bring anything into your life with dedication, thoughts of possibility, and hard work.

Passion for Life

"You've gotta dance like there's nobody watching,
Love like you'll never be hurt,
Sing like there's nobody listening,
And live like it's heaven on earth." ~William W. Purkey

Living a life that is *fully alive*, to me, means being passionate about everything I do, who I am, and how I hope to inspire others—both today and in the future. It also means keeping myself on the path and continuing to learn, grow, and strive to be the person I was intended to be... inside and out. In other words, choosing life every day!

There was a time when I didn't "choose life." I think back to that family trip we took to Mexico. It was supposed to be a trip to remember. We were in paradise, yet all I could see were the same things I saw and felt at home: physical pain, sadness, and resentment about not being able to do what I wanted to do.

I saw myself as a heavy woman who used to be athletic. I saw a woman in pain, one who had a hard time moving, let alone playing with her girls in the sand. I felt alone, sad, and in need of a hug, and spent my vacation time feeling sorry for myself. I yelled at my family and hardly stopped to enjoy a moment of it.

I remember that trip all right. But not for the reasons I should have: time with family, the beauty that surrounded us, fun times at the beach, or even the sunshine on our faces. Instead, I remember that week as a turning point for me. I didn't want to live on the sidelines of life any longer. I needed to live. Not just to exist, but to *live fully alive every day*.

Stop and truly think about what living fully alive means to you. Choose to live, grow, and become the best version of yourself today!

Breathe

Believe

Become

TAKE ACTION:
~YOUR STEPS FOR SUCCESS~

"We delight in the beauty of the butterfly, but rarely admit the changes it has gone through to achieve that beauty." ~Maya Angelou

The action steps in this section are for you, so you can take some time to sit down and really think about how you can put the concept of *Breathe, Believe, Become* into action. These steps will help you dive deeper and accomplish any positive goal you desire.

I encourage you to use a journal to take these action steps. You can also visit my website to print these steps out: **www.LiveAliveFit.com**

Set a date to complete the steps. Begin right away. By doing so, you will be giving yourself a huge gift: the gift of a great life.

It is time to begin **LIVING Your Best Life…Alive, Healthy, and Fit!**

1

ACTION STEP

TAKE
INVENTORY

Action Step: Inventory Your Primary and Secondary Foods

Take 15 minutes and write a few words about how you are feeling right now about each of the following areas of your life. As we discussed in the "Breathe" part of this book, these four areas are called Primary Food.

❋ Career

❋ Relationships

❋ Physical activity

❋ Spirituality

Get specific. "I am feeling bad about my weight right now" doesn't help define where you really are. Saying "I am four sizes larger than I would like to be" is specific.

When you accomplish the changes you choose to go after, you can later look back on this exercise, remember where you were, and celebrate the strength of the person who opened his or her heart to reveal what was inside.

Remember to be good to yourself and judgment-free.

❈ **Career:** *Whatever you have chosen to do at this time in your life, whether you are a stay-at-home parent, student, artist, volunteer, office worker, medical professional, or anything else, answer the following questions.*

◆ What have you chosen for your career?

◆ Are you in a career that you can't wait to get up in the morning for?

◆ Does your current career bring you energy and life?

◆ Does your career bring you the funds that you need to live?

◆ Are you passionate about what you do such that you can hardly believe you are getting paid to enjoy it?

◆ Share something that you have always dreamed of doing, but held yourself back from because of educational constraints, your age, your finances, or where you live.

❈ **Relationships:** *Our relationships with family, friends, partners, children, and co-workers shape our lives. Those we choose to surround ourselves with encourage, inspire, and love us, and they share joy, despair, and the experience of aging with us.*

◆ Do you live near and feel supported by your family?

◆ Do you have a partner or someone you can trust to call at any hour of the day or night with your most exciting wins or most challenging life moments?

◆ Do you spend time with friends physically in person—not just via the phone or Internet?

◆ Do you have children or wish you did?

◆ Are the people you work with each day people who bring you joy and happiness, or are they hard on you and make you feel less than you are?

◆ Are there people in your life whose entrance into a room makes you feel instantly better?

❋ **Physical Exercise:** *Movement of any kind can get our heart pumping while keeping our muscles and bones strong. Exercise gives us mental clarity and helps us sleep and recover faster. Movement can be anything from housework, to yard work, to a physical career, to daily or weekly workouts in a gym.*

◆ What types of exercise do you do each week?

◆ How long do you exercise within each workout time?

◆ Are you the type of person who gets your movement in preparing for and getting to work, along with housework?

◆ Are you taking additional time during the week to lift weights, take a walk, swim, enjoy a yoga class, run, ski, go cycling, or something else?

◆ Do you exercise at home, outside, or in a gym?

◆ Do you exercise with friends, family, or on your own?

◆ What type of exercise would you choose to do if you could fit it into your current schedule?

❋ **Spirituality:** *No matter what you believe in or how you bring it into your life, believing in something greater than yourself can clear your mind, allowing you to become more "present" in your day and bringing you a greater sense of inclusion in this world.*

◆ Do you participate in yoga, meditation, a walk in the park, or other activities that slow you down and bring you back into the present moment?

◆ Are you someone who attends church, mass, or another organized religious or spiritual service with family or friends?

◆ What would you choose to do—if you could make more time—to incorporate more quiet, reflective time into your life?

Nutrition: *Food = Fuel. How we choose to feed ourselves every day dictates how we feel and move through life. We often use food for more than just fueling our bodies, so we need to really think about why we are eating the things we eat. For this reason, we consider nutrition to be Secondary Food.*

◆ Are you eating for life, versus eating to compensate for emotions you wish you were feeling or to celebrate when something goes your way?

◆ Do you eat when you are bored?

◆ Do you drink, smoke, or add other things to your body that are unhealthy?

◆ What percent of your meals are home-cooked by you, a partner, or a family member?

◆ What would your meals and preparation time look like if you had all the time in the world to explore new options?

When you think about how you feel about each of these important areas of your life, you might find that one or two areas are not where you would like them to be. If so, ask yourself, what would you like to be different? The answer to this question is the perfect place to look at when creating and going after new goals.

2

ACTION STEP

DEFINE YOURSELF

Action Step: How Do You Want to Be Defined?

I remember the day I added "athlete" to my own "I AM" statement. It was not the day I completed my first race or even the day I could run three miles. It was the day I chose to start moving again and not let my injuries keep me from feeling alive.

Maybe there is something you would like to be defined by. Now is your chance to choose what that will be.

◆ What do you like being defined by from your past?

◆ What do you enjoy being defined by today?

◆ What would you like to be defined by in your future?

3

ACTION STEP

FIND YOUR PASSION

Action Step: What Are You Passionate About?

Take some time to think about the things that give you energy and passion in your life—things that you enjoy to such a degree that they don't even qualify as "real work." Things you might even do for free if you could.

Too many of us continue to do the same type of work year after year, not even considering whether it brings us joy and energy.

◆ What is something that you would cancel most anything in order to get to do?

◆ What is something that you would wake up early to do, even if you are not a morning person?

◆ Think of a time when you were doing an activity for a long stretch of time, and you were so lost in it with joy that you didn't even remember to stop and eat?

◆ When you even think of these activities, they make you smile:

◆ What are some activities or people you spend time with that give you energy instead of taking it away?

◆ What activity will you enjoy in the next seven days that gives you passion?

4

ACTION STEP

DREAM
DREAM DREAM

Action Step: Dream, Dream, Dream

Take some time to dream. Find a quiet place to sit where you feel comfortable and happy. Fetch a glass of water or cup of tea and take a deep breath.

Don't edit yourself, just let your thoughts flow and record what comes to your mind.

- ◆ When you were a child, what did you dream of doing?

- ◆ What types of things did you enjoy doing in the past that you no longer do? Did you used to play an instrument? Sew? Exercise? Think of things you cut out of your life when you became too "busy" to fit them in.

- ◆ Think of a time you shared your life with someone— maybe that's now. When you engage in more time with that person, do you eliminate things that once gave you joy in order to spend more time with them?

- ◆ When you daydream, what do you imagine yourself doing? Where do you imagine yourself living?

◆ If you were to be given millions of dollars—or enough to live on for a lifetime without ever having to work for money again—what would you do with your newly gained time?

◆ What goal could you create to move you closer to living the life of your dreams?

5

ACTION STEP

CREATE MEANING

Action Step: Create Meaning in Your Life

Give yourself some time to think about the things that add meaning to your life and bring it value. Remember, you can always add to your list as you keep this idea in mind over the next week.

◆ What do you think of when you imagine what your life means to others?

◆ How would others describe or define you?

◆ What does the opinion of others mean to you?

◆ What do you want to accomplish in your life?

◆ What adds value or meaning to your life?

◆ Are there ways that you would like to give back, either in support of others in their endeavors or by giving your time, money, or material goods?

◆ In the next seven days, what is one thing you can do to move you closer to living your life with meaning?

6

ACTION STEP

LONG-TERM
G O A L S

Action Step: Long-Term Goals

Take a moment to come up with a goal or two that you truly want to achieve this year. Think of goals that you would later regret not going after in, say, five years. Dream big; make it a bit uncomfortable to achieve. That is when you will rise to the occasion.

At the same time, make sure your goals are specific and measurable. Take the time to write down the details of when and how you will achieve your goals. Without specific dates and ways to measure your goals, there cannot be accountability. Be sure to use words that affirm what you will do. "I will..."

◆ What goal will you achieve in the next year?

Example: "I WILL become a total of 25 pounds lighter in six months. I currently weigh in at 190 pounds, and WILL reach 165 pounds." Or "In ten months, I WILL be able to walk 13.1 miles continuously."

◆ What day will you begin and what day will you complete your journey?

Example: "I WILL begin my goal on May 1st and I WILL accomplish my goal of becoming 25 pounds lighter by November first." Or "I will begin on May first, and by March first of next year, I WILL accomplish my goal of walking 13.1 miles without stopping at the half-marathon."

◆ What will you feel when you complete your goal?

Example: "WHEN I accomplish my goal I WILL not only feel healthier, but I WILL feel good in my own skin, take pride in how I look and feel, and believe that anything I set out to do, I can accomplish." Or *"I WILL realize my dream of completing a half-marathon, and I will get to do it with a friend."*

◆ What will you need to do to accomplish this goal?

Example: "I WILL eat three correctly portioned and healthy meals each day in addition to two or three healthy snacks, and I WILL exercise a minimum of three times a week for thirty to sixty minutes each time."

7

ACTION STEP

SHORT-TERM G O A L S

Action Step: Short-Term Goals

Take a moment to list the short-term goals that will ultimately enable you to achieve your long-term goal and keep you moving forward for the next few months. Make sure your short-term goals are specific. Just like your long-term goals, without specific dates and ways to measure your goals, there cannot be accountability.

This is where it gets serious. These are the goals that will keep you moving forward each and every day. Break down your larger goal into smaller goals that you know you need to reach in order to accomplish it.

For example, in my first triathlon I knew I needed to be able to do four things:

♦ Swim half a mile

♦ Ride a bike for 12 miles

♦ Run 3.1 miles

♦ And be able to do all these things, back to back, at once

I knew that I would need to practice each sport alone, and reach each individual milestone, but also be able to put them all together.

◆ What goal(s) will you achieve in the next two to four months that will get you closer to your long-term goal?

Example: "I WILL become 15 pounds lighter in three months. I currently weigh in at 190 pounds first thing in the morning, and I WILL weigh in at 175 pounds." Or "I WILL measure my strength according to how long I can walk in each workout. Currently I can walk for ten minutes, and in three months I will be able to walk nonstop for seventy minutes."

◆ On what day will you begin and complete your journey?

Example: "I WILL begin my goal on May first and accomplish my goals by August first."

◆ What will you feel when you complete your goal?

Example: "WHEN I accomplish my goal I will not only feel healthier and stronger, but I WILL feel good in my own skin, and not shy away from wearing summer clothing. This goal will also help me get one step closer to achieving my physical goal of walking a half-marathon by March of next year."

◆ What will you need to do to accomplish this goal?

Example: "I WILL add five minutes to the length of my walking time each week." Or "I WILL choose to eliminate all desserts, alcohol, and white flour carbohydrates from my meals, except for one meal a week." Or "I WILL make time in my daily schedule to get my workouts in."

8

ACTION STEP

LIFE GOALS & INTENTIONS

Action Step: Life Goals and Intentions

Please take some time to stop and think about how you hope to live your life. What do you want your legacy to be? What brings you joy and energy?

With these ideas in mind, take the time to write down a few things that resonate with the way you ultimately want to live in order to be your true self. These are not necessarily things that you are doing today, but things that represent who you want to be, and ways you could live each day in order to grow closer to the life that you are intended to live. For an example of my life goals and intentions, refer back the "Small Steps Turn into Giant Leaps" chapter in the "Breathe" section.

- ◆ What life goals and intentions do you want to live out each day?

- ◆ What life goals and intentions do you hope to live by this year?

Once you've created this list, print it out to see each day. Note that your written-down life goals and intentions will always be a working document. Please do not feel pressured to decide your entire future today. My list of life goals and intentions has evolved many times since I first wrote it down years ago.

You will want to come back to this list from time to time. It can be every six months, once a year, or longer, but every once in a while, check to see if your intentions are still in line with the way you are choosing to live your life. This will give you overall direction along your newly created life path.

9

ACTION STEP

TAKING TIME
FOR ME

Action Step: I Am Worth the Time I Take for Me

Once you have your short-term, long-term, and life goals written down, take a close look at how you are spending your time. This will give you some insight into how you could spend your time more efficiently and make the time to do the things that will get you closer to your goals. This will give you more excitement and energy for each day.

- ◆ Make a list of all the things that you do every day for a week. Write down everything, even simple chores. Include the time you spend cleaning and maintaining your home, working, commuting, exercising, taking care of children, volunteering, watching TV, reading books, going to school, etc. Then tally up your time spent on each task to find out how many minutes or hours a week you spend doing each thing.

- ◆ Make particular note of the things you do on weekends or days off, including how long you spend doing them every week.

- ◆ Make a list of all the things you do for fun for a few weeks, and how long you spend doing them.

Now, take a look at your lists of things. Label each with the words "Need," "Want," "Others," and "Take" according to the below rules. Note that some items will have more than one label.

◆ Label the items that you <u>NEED</u> to continue to do to, like working, taking care of your children, grocery shopping, cleaning your home, etc.

◆ Label the items that you <u>WANT</u> to continue to do because they bring you joy and happiness and make you feel alive, like practicing yoga, hanging out with friends, watching a certain amount of television, spending time on social media, cooking at home, reading before bed, etc.

◆ Label the items that you do for <u>OTHERS</u> because you feel obligated, like carpooling, volunteering at school, etc.

◆ Now look back through the entire list and label the items that you notice <u>TAKE</u> energy away from you. These are things that you do each week that drag you down and drain your mental energy—things you find yourself trying to avoid, like cleaning the bathroom, getting up early to drive to work, completing paperwork, etc.

Without taking the time to look at your priorities, you might not have realized how draining some parts of your week are. Could you choose to change things around to add more value and brighten your week? By eliminating some of the things that take energy away from you, you will create time to fit in workouts, learn a new skill, go back to school, or achieve any other goal that you set for yourself.

10

ACTION STEP

AM I
READY?

Action Step: Am I Ready?

Take a moment to answer the following questions from your heart. These are big questions, but I know you are ready to answer them. Being self-aware enough to make these tough decisions will help you accomplish any goal.

If these questions are challenging for you, then you are on the right track. If they were easy to answer you would have already achieved your goals. There has been something that has held you back from each of them. Now is the time to discover what that *something* is for you and move past it in order to truly live.

◆ Are you ready to take the leap and go after your dreams?

◆ When will your desire to achieve your goals outweigh the pain of staying the same? Is that time now?

◆ If not, what would have to align for you to trust yourself and go for it?

11

ACTION STEP

WHY,

WHY?

Action Step: Why, WHY?

Even more important than having your goal in front of you is having the personal reasons why you will accomplish it. Never lose sight of these reasons. This exercise will help you clarify your reasons for wanting to accomplish your goal.

◆ Why do you want to accomplish your goal?

◆ What benefits will come to you when you accomplish it?

◆ What will it feel like to succeed?

◆ How will you feel one year from now if you choose not to go after your goal?

◆ How will you feel five years from now if you choose not to go after your goal?

12

ACTION STEP

YOUR ENVIRONMENT

Action Step: Your Environment

Take some time to answer the questions below to give you a better sense of your current environment: who you hang out with, and where. Your environment is an important factor in supporting you and helping you move closer to being the best person you can be, so you want to make sure it is clean and full of possibility!

◆ Do your friends always want to meet in locations that reinforce unhealthy behavior you are working to change? For instance, do they often want to meet at bars and clubs, even though you are trying to stay away from alcohol? Where could you suggest going to that would be in line with your new healthy life?

◆ Do you have a friend or spouse that frequently wants to go out to dinner or stop for quick meals at restaurants? Or does your partner cook or encourage you to cook healthy meals and enjoy sitting together for a nice quiet meal? If not, would you be willing to encourage them to cook with you a few times a week instead of going out?

◆ Do you currently spend time with a friend that you feel doesn't have your best interests in mind, for instance, someone who constantly wants to go shopping even though you are on a very strict budget? Where could you suggest meeting that would be in line with your new lifestyle?

◆ Does your workplace support the choices you make to live your best life? For instance, does it have a shower or changing room so you can exercise or walk during lunch? Or does everyone in your office take smoke breaks so that you feel obligated to join them in order to feel included? Are there candy dishes on the reception desk that you walk by daily, undermining your goal of becoming twenty pounds lighter? Where could you go during lunch or a break to realign yourself with your goals (e.g. walk to a park, visit a museum, go to the gym, or write in a journal)?

◆ What types of activities would you like to be doing that you currently are not, but that you would if you had friends to do them with? For instance, I used to play soccer every week with friends, but once I moved, I no longer had that same support group, so I stopped playing soccer. Where could you find a group of people who enjoy similar interests (e.g. at work, through social networking, by asking friends)?

◆ Who do you currently spend time with that makes you feel great? Could you spend more time with them?

13

ACTION STEP

CONQUER
FEAR

Action Step: Conquer Your Fear

Take some time to think about what might be holding you back from accomplishing your goals. What ideas in your head are stopping you in your tracks, making it seemingly impossible for you to move forward?

◆ When you think about achieving your goal, what feelings immediately come to mind?

◆ What or from whom do you feel the most resistance when you attempt certain tasks to help you accomplish your goal?

◆ This week, in what ways will you choose to stare your fears in the eye and walk straight toward them, despite any uncomfortable feelings, to help you get closer to accomplishing your goal?

◆ How good will it feel when you overcome the feelings of resistance and do what you need to do in order to live your best life by going after your goal?

14

ACTION STEP

PLAN
AHEAD

Action Step: Plan Ahead

Having too large of goals can make some of us more likely to quit, so make sure you take your short-term goals and break them down into manageable weekly and daily tasks. This creates momentum that you can use to achieve your complete goal. By answering the questions below, you will set yourself up for success.

Every Sunday night, take some time to create a list of tasks for the week ahead. By doing so, not only will you be more organized, but you will also be able to avoid last-minute changes that could cut into the time that you had set aside for your goal.

◆ What do I need to do tomorrow, and each day this week, to move me closer to my goal?

◆ What do I need to do by the end of the week to move me closer to my goal?

◆ What can I do ahead of time to ensure that I get the time I need to accomplish my goal in a timely manner and hold my commitment to myself?

15

ACTION STEP

I

A M

Action Step: I AM...

Take a moment to center yourself in a quiet space. Clear your mind and take a few deep cleansing breaths. Remember a time when you accomplished something you deemed amazing. I am sure it wasn't easy to accomplish that goal, but you did it.

Now I want you to open your eyes and write down anything that comes into your mind. Don't edit yourself. Just let the words flow in any order and in any place on your page.

◆ Write words that make you feel great. "I am..."

◆ Write words that resonate with who you will become. "I will be..."

◆ Write words that you know deep inside are true to you. "I am..."

Look at the list you've made. This is who you truly ARE and who you WILL fully become when you choose to believe it. This is where it gets exciting. The power we have over our minds is so incredible, you just need to harness it. Create an "I AM..." statement now that reflects all of the things you are. For an example, mine is below.

I AM... Mary! Wife, Mother, Sister, Daughter, Aunt, Friend, Athlete, Artist, Speaker, Author, Student of Life, Inspiration for All... Caring, Passionate, Loving, Compassionate, Grateful. I AM HEALTHY and STRONG to live the life I know I can!

16

ACTION STEP

WHAT
YOU LOVE

Action Step: What Do You Love?

Set a timer for five or ten minutes and write down all of the things that you love. Some are obvious, some simple, and some are more subtle, but they are all important and give great joy and love.

Use this exercise any time you need to be uplifted. It can be done verbally (best if said out loud) or in writing. Give it a try—you will be grinning from ear to ear before this exercise is over. If not, keep going. Love brings love.

◆ "I love..."

◆ "I love..."

◆ "I love..."

17

ACTION STEP

PASSION FOR LIFE

Action Step: Passion for Life

Take some time to stop and truly think about what *Living Fully Alive* means to you. What does it include?

This can be a work in progress, evolving as you do. Keep it nearby so that you can adjust it as you grow and become the best version of yourself.

◆ What does Living Fully Alive mean to you?

◆ How does it correlate to your life goals?

Notes

With gratitude for their generous permission to quote from their works, the author acknowledges the following resources:

1 IRONMAN® and IRONMAN® 70.3®, and their respective logos, are registered trademarks of World Triathlon Corporation in the United States and other countries. This independent publication has not been authorized, endorsed, sponsored, or licensed by, nor has content been reviewed or otherwise approved by, World Triathlon Corporation dba IRONMAN®

2 The terms "Primary Food" and "Secondary Food" are trademarks that are owned by Integrative Nutrition Inc. (used under license).

3 http://www.merriam-webster.com/dictionary/carpe%20diem

4 http://en.wikipedia.org/wiki/Four-minute_mile

5 The War Of Art, Steven Pressfield, page 12. Copyright 2002 Black Irish Entertainment. All rights reserved.

6 http://www.merriam-webster.com/dictionary/love

7 http://themindunleashed.org/2014/01/scientific-proof-thoughts-intentions-can-alter-physical-world-around-us.html

Excited About Living Your Best Life?

My true passion is helping others find their path in life. Join me at www.LiveAliveFit.com to receive more information about "Living Your Best Life… Alive, Healthy & Fit." There you will find information about one-on-one and group coaching in health, nutrition, fitness, and yoga. You can also sign up to receive my newsletters and information on upcoming speaking engagements.

I can help you sort through your dreams, create meaningful goals, and give you the accountability you need to accomplish them. I can't wait to help you become the person you were meant to be. To book me to speak at your workplace or special event, or for an initial health history consultation, reach me on the web at **www.LiveAliveFit.com**. What are you waiting for? Contact me today!

Already living a life you desire? I received my Health Coaching Certification at the Institute of Integrative Nutrition. If you are interested in health, nutrition, and wellness (like I am), you will love their amazing online program. It teaches a holistic and bio-individual approach to health. For more information about nutrition, health coaching, or The Institute of Integrative Nutrition—or have any specific questions about the program—I would love to connect at **www.LiveAliveFit.com**.

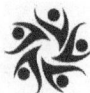

About the Author

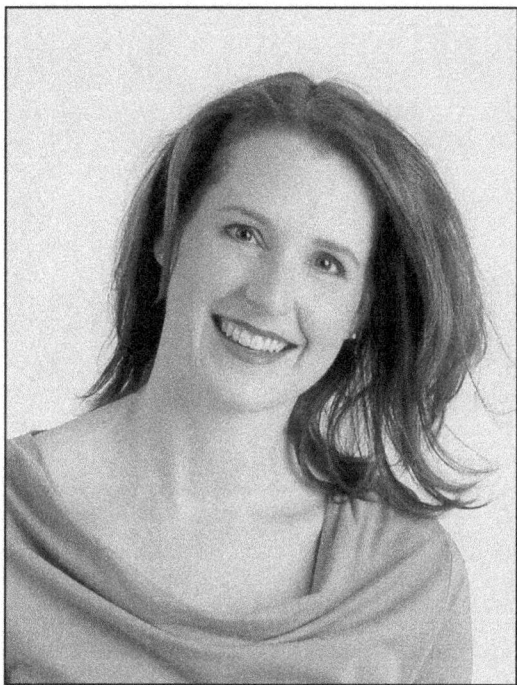

Mary Caroline Craig is a Certified Integrative Health, Nutrition, and Fitness Coach as well as a speaker and author. She guides her clients to "Live their Best Lives...Alive, Healthy, and Fit." She is a member of the Team USA ITU Age Group World Duathlon Championship team, a competitive triathlete, a multisport coach, a Certified Yoga Instructor, a mother, and a learner for life. Mary, along with her two lovely daughters and husband, resides in beautiful Seattle, WA. You can reach her on the web at **www.LiveAliveFit.com** and on Facebook at: www.facebook.com/livealivefit.